CANCER ETIOLOGY, DIAGNOSIS AND TREATMENTS

COLORECTAL CANCER

PREVENTION, DIAGNOSIS AND TREATMENT

CANCER ETIOLOGY, DIAGNOSIS AND TREATMENTS

Additional books and e-books in this series can be found on Nova's website under the Series tab.

CANCER ETIOLOGY, DIAGNOSIS AND TREATMENTS

COLORECTAL CANCER

PREVENTION, DIAGNOSIS AND TREATMENT

MASAYOSHI YAMAGUCHI
EDITOR

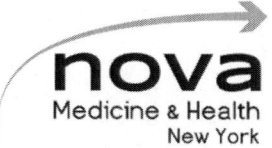

Copyright © 2020 by Nova Science Publishers, Inc.

All rights reserved. No part of this book may be reproduced, stored in a retrieval system or transmitted in any form or by any means: electronic, electrostatic, magnetic, tape, mechanical photocopying, recording or otherwise without the written permission of the Publisher.

We have partnered with Copyright Clearance Center to make it easy for you to obtain permissions to reuse content from this publication. Simply navigate to this publication's page on Nova's website and locate the "Get Permission" button below the title description. This button is linked directly to the title's permission page on copyright.com. Alternatively, you can visit copyright.com and search by title, ISBN, or ISSN.

For further questions about using the service on copyright.com, please contact:
Copyright Clearance Center
Phone: +1-(978) 750-8400 Fax: +1-(978) 750-4470 E-mail: info@copyright.com.

NOTICE TO THE READER

The Publisher has taken reasonable care in the preparation of this book, but makes no expressed or implied warranty of any kind and assumes no responsibility for any errors or omissions. No liability is assumed for incidental or consequential damages in connection with or arising out of information contained in this book. The Publisher shall not be liable for any special, consequential, or exemplary damages resulting, in whole or in part, from the readers' use of, or reliance upon, this material. Any parts of this book based on government reports are so indicated and copyright is claimed for those parts to the extent applicable to compilations of such works.

Independent verification should be sought for any data, advice or recommendations contained in this book. In addition, no responsibility is assumed by the Publisher for any injury and/or damage to persons or property arising from any methods, products, instructions, ideas or otherwise contained in this publication.

This publication is designed to provide accurate and authoritative information with regard to the subject matter covered herein. It is sold with the clear understanding that the Publisher is not engaged in rendering legal or any other professional services. If legal or any other expert assistance is required, the services of a competent person should be sought. FROM A DECLARATION OF PARTICIPANTS JOINTLY ADOPTED BY A COMMITTEE OF THE AMERICAN BAR ASSOCIATION AND A COMMITTEE OF PUBLISHERS.

Additional color graphics may be available in the e-book version of this book.

Library of Congress Cataloging-in-Publication Data

ISBN: 978-1-53616-598-2
Library of Congress Control Number:2019953055

Published by Nova Science Publishers, Inc. † New York

CONTENTS

Preface		vii
Chapter 1	The Inhibitory Effect of Polysaccharides on Colorectal Cancer *Yan Lu and Kaoshan Chen*	1
Chapter 2	The Role of Regucalcin as a Suppressor in Human Colorectal Cancer *Masayoshi Yamaguchi*	31
Chapter 3	An Aryl Hydrocarbon Receptor Agonist Suppresses the Growth of Human Colorectal Cancer Cells *Masayoshi Yamaguchi*	51
Chapter 4	Surgical Approach to Rectal Cancer *Jelena Petrovic Sunderic*	67
About the Editor		93
Index		95
Related Nova Publications		103

PREFACE

Carcinogenesis is a multistep process initiated by external stimuli that lead to genetic changes in normal cells or stem cells, resulting in proliferation, apoptosis, dysplasia and neoplasia. The expression, post-translational processing, and targeting of the gene products are frequently altered in transformed and malignant cells. Currently, prognosis of advanced cancer remains poor in spite of the development of novel therapeutic strategies. Improved knowledge of the oncogenic processes and signaling pathways that regulate tumor cell proliferation, differentiation, angiogenesis, invasion and metastasis has led to the identification of several potential therapeutic targets, which have driven the development of molecularly targeted therapies. The target is "drugable" as an enzyme (kinase) or cell surface molecule (membrane-bound receptors) that can be easily screened for small-molecule inhibitors or targeted by a specific antibody. New perspectives in cancer treatment have appeared with the advent of microRNAs, a novel class of noncoding small RNAs. Moreover, identification of the genes that are differentially expressed between sensitive and resistant cancer cells for chemotherapy and radiation is important in the ability to predict the clinical effectiveness of therapy and develop the new therapeutic tool.

Adenocarcinoma is the predominant malignancy found in the colon and rectum. Colorectal cancer is the third most common cancer diagnosed in the developed world with a high incidence of mortality and morbidity. The average 5-year survival rate remains poor at 55%, although the development of new drugs has improved the survival rate of colorectal cancer patients. The prognosis of colorectal cancer remains poor in spite of the development of novel therapeutic strategies. Human colorectal cancer represents a heterogeneous group of diseases, and its molecular classification is increasingly important. Characterization of novel biomarker targets may lead to prolong the survival of colorectal cancer. Biomarkers may have a potential role in screening, diagnosis, prognosis and monitoring disease. Mutations in the *KRAS* gene in ~ 40% of tumors have been reported to be induced by genetic and epigenetic alterations. This book introduces the recent topics regarding colorectal cancer, and provides the recent highlighted information concerning prevention, diagnosis and treatment, and it is constituted of chapter 1-4, as summarized in the following.

Chapter 1 reviews the inhibitory effect of polysaccharides on colorectal cancer. Colorectal cancer is one of the most common malignancies and one of the leading causes of cancer-related deaths worldwide, and effective therapies are urgently needed to control human colorectal cancer. However, surgery, chemotherapy, radiotherapy and the chemotherapy drugs currently on the market have various side effects to reduce the quality of life of patients. Fortunately, many natural polysaccharides have been extracted from fungi, plants, animal, algae, and lichens, and these polysaccharides have been found to possess anti-colon cancer activities and prevention of colon cancer or can increase the efficacy of conventional chemotherapy drugs though a variety of mechanisms. *In vivo* and *in vitro* experiments have demonstrated that the anti-colon cancer activity of polysaccharides is mainly shown in activating the PI3K/Akt, NF-κB, MAPK, P53, and AMPK signaling pathway, inducing colon cancer cell mitochondrial apoptosis, or cycle arrest, inhibiting colon cancer cell metastasis, influencing the inflammatory response and regulating the gut microflora. Based on these encouraging observations, many researches have been focused on discovering anti-colon cancer polysaccharides. Therefore, our research team launched a comprehensive review to summarize the studies reported last decades and our research progress. However, these polysaccharides were tested using the cells and animal models, few were involved in clinical studies. This chapter increases our understanding of the anti-colon cancer activities of polysaccharides and related signaling pathway. It will be helpful in developing and designing more effectively anti-colon cancer drugs.

Chapter 2 proposes a potential role of regucalcin as a suppressor gene in human colorectal cancer. Regucalcin plays a crucial role as a regulator of transcription signaling activity, and its lowered expression or activity may contribute in the promotion of human carcinogenesis. Higher regucalcin expression in the tumor tissues has been demonstrated to prolong survival of patients with cancer of various types, including pancreatic cancer, breast cancer, liver cancer, and lung adenocarcinoma. The involvement of regucalcin in human colorectal cancer was investigated in the current study. The regucalcin gene expression and survival data of 62 patients were obtained though the Gene Expression Omnibus (GEO) database (GSE12945), to analysis outcome. Data of gene expression showed that prolonged survival in colorectal cancer patients is associated with higher regucalcin gene expression in tumor tissues. Overexpression of regucalcin depressed colony formation, proliferation and death of human colorectal carcinoma RKO cells *in vitro*. Mechanistically, overexpressed regucalcin induced G1 and G2/M phase cell cycle arrest of RKO cells through suppression of multiple signaling pathways including Ras, Akt, MAP kinase and SAPK/JNK. Interestingly, overexpressed regucalcin caused elevation of the tumor suppressers p53 and Rb, and cell cycle inhibitor p21. Moreover, c-*fos*, c-jun, NF-κB p65, β-catenin, and Stat3, transcription factor, were repressed by overexpressed regucalcin. This study suggests that regucalcin plays a crucial role as a suppressor in human colorectal cancer, and that the suppressed regucalcin gene expression may predispose patients to the promotion of colorectal cancer. Overexpressed regucalcin with the gene delivery may play a role as a novel therapy of colorectal cancer.

Chapter 3 introduces the recent topics that an arylhydrocarbone receptor agonist suppresses the growth human colorectal cancer cells. Human colorectal cancer, which represents a heterogenous group of diseases, is the third most common cancer with the average 5-year survival rate at 55%. Characterization of novel biomarker targets with molecular classification may lead to prolonging survival of colorectal cancer. The aryl hydrocarbon receptor (AHR) is transcriptionally active in the form of a heterodimer with the AHR nuclear translocator, which then binds to the xenobiotic responsive element. AHR was initially discovered via its ligand, the polychlorinated hydrocarbon, 2,3,7,8-tetrachlorodibenzo-p-dioxin (TCDD). We investigated whether TCDD, an agonist of AHR signaling, regulates the growth of RKO human colorectal cancer cells *in vitro*. Treatment with TCDD (0.1-100 nM) revealed suppressive effects on colony formation and proliferation of RKO cells, and stimulated death of these cells with subconfluence. These effects of TCDD were abolished by pretreatment with CH223191, an inhibitor of AHR signaling. Western blot analysis showed that TCDD treatment decreased AHR levels and elevated CYP1A1 levels, indicating a stimulation of AHR signaling. TCDD treatment caused the increase in NF-κB p65 and β-catenin, although it did not have an effect on Ras levels. Importantly, TCDD treatment increased the levels of p53, Rb, p21, and regucalcin, which are suppressors of the growth of tumor cells. Of note, effects of TCDD on the proliferation and death were not revealed in regucalcin-overexpressing RKO cells, and regucalcin overexpression depressed AHR signaling linked to CYP1A1 expression. Thus, AHR signaling suppresses the growth of colorectal cancer cells, suggesting a role as a novel targeting molecule for colorectal cancer.

Chapter 4 highlights the surgical approach to rectal cancer. Until recently surgery was the only mean of rectal cancer treatment and was not entirely successful in advanced cases. The development of the oncologic agents and radiotherapeutic approaches have given justified hope even for those patients. Nevertheless, the principles of surgery have remained the same, since so far achieved "gold standard" in rectal cancer surgery, based on total mesorectal excision within the strict anatomic borders, has shown the best immediate and late postoperative results, quality of life and the lowest recurrence rate. New technologies, like laparoscopic and robotic surgeries, are not offering oncologic benefits compared to the open approach, but have immediate postoperative advances. They are getting more widely accepted both by the surgeons and patients, but are still on trial due to specific considerations. Apart from the radical surgeries, in some cases palliative procedures are unavoidable, and the aforementioned new oncological advancements can convert inoperable into operable cases.

As introduced above, this book focuses recent topics on prevention, diagnosis and treatment implicated in colorectal cancer. The editor believes that this book will be of interest to undergraduate and graduate students, biomedical researchers, and medical doctors focused on the fields of molecular and cellular biology, medical sciences, and clinical challenges.

Editor
Masayoshi Yamaguchi, PhD, IOM, FAOE, DDG, DG
University of Hawaii Cancer Center,
University of Hawaii at Manoa,
Honolulu, Hawaii, USA

In: Colorectal Cancer ISBN: 978-1-53616-598-2
Editor: Masayoshi Yamaguchi © 2020 Nova Science Publishers, Inc.

Chapter 1

THE INHIBITORY EFFECT OF POLYSACCHARIDES ON COLORECTAL CANCER

Yan Lu and Kaoshan Chen[*]
School of Life Science, Shandong University, Qingdao, China

ABSTRACT

Colorectal cancer is one of the most common malignancies and one of the leading causes of cancer-related deaths worldwide, and effective therapies are urgently needed to control human colorectal cancer. However, surgery, chemotherapy, radiotherapy and the chemotherapy drugs currently on the market have various side effects to reduce the quality of life of patients. Fortunately, many natural polysaccharides have been extracted from fungi, plants, animal, algae, and lichens, and these polysaccharides have been found to possess anti-colon cancer activities and prevention of colon cancer or can increase the efficacy of conventional chemotherapy drugs though a variety of mechanisms. *In vivo* and *in vitro* experiments have demonstrated that the anti-colon cancer activity of polysaccharides is mainly shown in activating the PI3K/Akt, NF-κB, MAPK, P53, and AMPK signaling pathway, inducing

---

[*] Corresponding Author's E-mail: ksc313@126.com.

colon cancer cell mitochondrial apoptosis, or cycle arrest, inhibiting colon cancer cell metastasis, influencing the inflammatory response and regulating the gut microflora. Based on these encouraging observations, many researches have been focused on discovering anti-colon cancer polysaccharides. Therefore, our research team launched a comprehensive review to summarize the studies reported last decades and our research progress. However, these polysaccharides were tested using the cells and animal models, few were involved in clinical studies. This chapter increases our understanding of the anti-colon cancer activities of polysaccharides and related signaling pathway. It will be helpful in developing and designing more effectively anti-colon cancer drugs.

Keywords: corolectal cancer, polysaccharide

OVERVIEW OF COLON CANCER

Colon Cancer Epidemiology

Colon cancer, also called colorectal cancer, is one of the common gastrointestinal malignant tumor, which can occur from the cecum to any part of the rectum and most often occurs at the junction of the rectum and sigmoid colon.

It is mainly caused by the abnormal proliferation of intestinal mucosal epithelial cells, which has the ability of invasion and proliferation and seriously threaten human health [1]. According to the world health organization statistics show that colon cancer is the third most common cancer in developed countries, as the change of diets and lifestyles, the incidence and mortality of colon cancer has been rising steadily in recent years [2]. The early symptom of colon cancer is insidious, often without any obvious clinical manifestations, to discover harder, causing tumor metastasis, therefore, patients would miss the optimal period of operation treatment [3].

Risk Factors for Colon Cancer

The development of colon cancer is not an isolated process, but a disease caused by the accumulation of multiple steps: The first stage is mainly manifested as the gene mutation of DNA damage caused by proliferation or uncontrollable abnormal proliferation of colon crypt cells; In the second stage, mutations in genes (proto-oncogene and cancer suppressor gene) that control the cell cycle leads to clonal amplification; Subsequently, the intraepithelial tumor spread to multiple sites in the colonic mucosa, leading to adenomatous polyps in the premalignant and premalignant stages.

However, tumor cells could become aggressive through crossing the epithelial basement membrane into other tissues. The occurrence and development of colon cancer is influenced by various factors, such as environment factor, genetic factor and host individual characteristic [3]. The etiology of colon cancer mainly includes traditional epidemiology and molecular epidemiology.

Traditional epidemiology is mainly limited to the external environment (bad dietary habits, such as high fat low fiber diet, animal protein, food nitrosamines and their derivatives high content, alcohol intake) and previous disease history [4]. High-fat diet leads to an increase in bile acids in the colon, which in turn causes anaerobic microorganisms (particularly carboxylic acid bacteria) to break down primary bile acids into secondary bile acids. Furthermore, the lack of fiber in the diet will also be a risk factor for colon cancer. Fiber can reduce the incidence of colon cancer by the following factors:

The generated short-chain fatty acids reduce pH to create an environment that is not conducive to the growth of cancer cells; Increased fecal volume to dilute colon carcinogen; Adsorption of bile salts, etc. In terms of lifestyle, poor bowel habits cause harmful substances to accumulate in the colon, thus damaging the intestinal mucosa and causing cancer. In addition, it is estimated that about 30% of colon cancer is related to genetic element, such as familial adenomatous polyposis and hereditary nonpolyposis colorectal cancer [5].

At the molecular level, the pathogenesis of the molecular mechanism of the development of colon cancer mainly includes the following aspects: Inactivation and functional loss of tumor suppressor genes (p53, APC, DCC, MCC gene) [3]; Overexpression and activation of proto-oncogenes (scr, and ras family); Mutations in repair genes [3]; Changes in telomerase length; Abnormal activation of relevant signaling pathways; Related apoptosis regulation disorder, and so on. The activation of proto-oncogenes causes the up-regulation of proliferation-related factors (CyclinA1, CyclinD1, CDK4, MST1) in tumor cells, while the inactivation of tumor suppressor genes induces uncontrolled growth of cells, makes the cancer cells not controlled by the body's defense system, and promotes the unlimited proliferation of tumor cells [6].

Prevention and Treatment of Colon Cancer

At present, the treatment principle of colorectal cancer is a comprehensive treatment based on surgery. Resection of the tumor is the most common and effective method for the treatment of colorectal cancer. Postoperative chemotherapy, radiotherapy, traditional Chinese medicine, immunotherapy and other means. For colon cancer with advanced metastatic or postoperative recurrence and metastasis, chemical drugs are particularly important [7]. Currently, the commonly used chemical drugs in clinical practice include alkylating agents, anti-metabolism, anti-tumor antibiotics, anti-tumor animal and plant ingredients drugs, anti-tumor hormones, and miscellaneous drugs. Furthermore, there are also new biological targeted agents, including epidermal growth factor receptor inhibitors and vascular endothelial factor inhibitors.

These drugs suppress the proliferation of cancer cells by interfering with the synthesis of DNA and RNA in the body. However, the chemotherapy drugs have some side effects, including dry mouth, loss of appetite, nausea, vomiting, sometimes appear oral mucosal inflammation or ulceration and bone marrow suppression, immunosuppression, liver damage, lung toxicity, kidney toxicity, heart toxicity, neurotoxicity, hair loss, etc. which seriously reduces the life quality of patients. In recent years, with the emergence of new tumor drugs and new targeted agents, the treatment of colon cancer has been significantly improved, while the early diagnosis rate of colon cancer in China is only 10-15%, and the survival rate of advanced colon cancer has not decreased. Therefore, the precaution of colon cancer becomes particularly important.

Nowadays, the prevention of colon cancer can be interfered from the following aspects: dietary adjustment, chemoprophylaxis, the treatment of precancerous lesions, screening of high-risk groups. Colon cancer already became a kind of "contemporary disease", and greatly related to the lifestyle of modern and dietary habit, especially high protein and tall adipose food, which causes excessive intake of energy. Conversely, increased prandial composition processed protective effect to colon cancer in daily diet, including dietary fiber, vitamin, microelement and unsaturated fatty acid, have active effect to preventing colon cancer. Chemoprophylaxis refers to the use of natural or synthetic chemical agents to prevent the occurrence of tumors [8]. According to the reports, the chemical drugs possessed prophylactic effect to colon cancer mainly have aspirin and other steroidal anti-inflammatory drug, folic acid, calcium, estrogen, vitamin and antioxidant. In addition, the treatment of precancerous lesions and screening of high groups can also play a good role in the prevention of colon cancer.

Overview of Polysaccharides

Research Progress of Polysaccharides

The study for sugar began in the mid-19th century, when Rasemacher, Parekh and Dwek at Oxford University published a paper entitled "Glycobiology" in 1988, which announced the official birth of "Glycobiology". Polysaccharides are natural polymers with complex structure, widely existing in plants, animals, microorganisms, algae and lichens [9]. Polysaccharides possess diverse biological activities, such as anti-tumor [10], immune-enhancing effect [11], antioxidant [12], antibacterial [8], anti-inflammatory [13], lipid-lowering and hypoglycemic [14], liver protection [15] and other pharmacological activities. The development and utilization of polysaccharides are attached great importance in China, lentinan [16], ginseng polysaccharides [17], griflola frondosa polysaccharide [18], coriolus versicolor polysaccharide [19] applied in clinical tumor treatment. Therefore, polysaccharides have broad application prospects in the fields of biochemistry, medicine and food development. It is undeniable that the research and development of active polysaccharides will become an important subject in life science.

The Mechanisms of Polysaccharides against Colon Cancer

Radiotherapy, chemotherapy and chemotherapy drugs possesses toxic side effects, thus causing a serious decline in the quality of life for colon cancer patients. In addition, surgical resection combined with adjuvant therapy is effective in the early stages of colon cancer, however, the recurrence and metastasis often occur [20]. Therefore, it is necessary to develop novel, high effective, low-toxicity or non-toxic drugs from natural chemicals to treat colon cancer. At present, a large number of *in vitro* and *in vivo* experiments have confirmed that polysaccharide extract has the effects of suppressing the proliferation of colon cancer cells and inducing the apoptosis of tumor cells [1]. The action mechanism of polysaccharides against colon cancer cell proliferation will be explained from the following aspects:

Mitochondrial Apoptotic Pathway

Mitochondria are the center of intracellular oxidative phosphorylation, the control hub of cell life activities and the important site of cell apoptosis regulation, and the target of various apoptosis signaling molecules [21]. Mitochondrial apoptosis is divided into endogenous mitochondrial apoptosis pathway and exogenous mitochondrial apoptosis pathway. In many cell types, the activation of the exogenous pathway can ensure the implementation of apoptosis in the mitochondrial pathway [22]. Suo et al. studied the inhibitory effect of polysaccharide of Larimichthys croces swim bladder (PLCSB) on human colon cancer cells (HCT-116). The results showed that PLCSB significantly up-regulated the expression level of Bax, p53, p21, caspase-3, caspase-8, caspase-9, Fas and apoptotic protease activating factor 1, and down-regulated the expression level of Bcl-2 [23]. Soy soluble polysaccharide (SSPS) have a variety of pharmacological effects, such as anti-inflammatory and immunomodulatory activities. KO et al. demonstrated that SPSS induced HCT-116 cell apoptosis, which relates to the generation of ROS, the damage of mitochondrial, the activator of caspase family, and the lysis of polymerase protein 2. In addition, SPSS decreased Bcl-2 expression and increased Bax and Bad expression [24]. Foreign scholar Ana et al. reported that polysaccharides from Common Beans (*Phaseolus vulgaris* L.) (PE) could alleviate AOM-induced colon cancer, which increases the concentration of short chain fatty acids in cecum, decreased the number of aberrant crypt, and induced up-regulation of Rb gene expression and down-regulation of Bax and caspase-3 gene expression [25]. SLNT, a water-soluble polysaccharide from *Lentinus edodes*, inhibits human colon cancer cell (HT-29) proliferation by mitochondrial apoptosis pathway. SLNT activates caspase-3, caspase-8, caspase-9, up-regulates cytochrome C expression and the ratio of Bax/Bcl-2, down-regulates the expression level of NF-κB, and the excess production of ROS and TNF-α [26]. Chinese scholar Liang et al. found that *Ganoderma lucidum* polysaccharides (GLPs) target a Fas/caspase dependent pathway to inhibit the proliferation and migration in human colon cancer cells (LoVo), and activate caspase-8, caspase-3 and up-regulate Fas expression to induce apoptosis in HCT-116 cells [27].

NF-κB Signaling

Nuclear transcription factor (NF-κB) is a key endogenous tumor promoter with a variety of cellular activities and play a vital role in integrating multiple stress stimuli and regulating inflammatory states in innate and adaptive immune responses. There are two main activator pathways: classical (dominated by p50/RelA-p65 heterodimer) and non-classical (composed of p52/RelB heterodimer) NF-κB signaling pathways [28]. Some data have suggested that polysaccharides can inhibit the proliferation of colon cancer cells by interfering with the translocation of NF-κB. Cheng and other researchers found that BP-1, a water-soluble polysaccharide was extracted from *highland barley*, consisted of glucose, xylose, arabinose, and rhamnose with the ratio of 8.82:1.92:1.50:1.00, with an average molecular weight of 6.7×10^4 Da. BP-1 induced HT-29 cell apoptosis by enhancing the phosphorylation of JNK, facilitating the production of ROS, and inhibiting the transfer of NF-κB from the cytoplasm to the nucleus. Meanwhile, BP-1-induced apoptosis is related to apoptosis-related proteins, such as Bcl-2, the release of cytochrome C from mitochondria to cytoplasm, and the activation of caspase-8 and caspase-9. These results showed that BP-1 induced apoptosis by the ROS-JNK and NF-κB-regulated caspase pathways [29]. Astragalus polysaccharide (APS) is a kind of astragalus extract with a wide range of medicinal values, including anti-inflammatory, antioxidant, anti-tumor and anti-diabetes effects. Lv et al. confirmed that APS significantly improved DSS-induced colitis by reducing the phosphorylation of NF-κB DNA, down-regulating the expression of TNF-α, IL-1β, IL-6, IL-17, and decreasing the activity of peroxidase [30]. Yue et al. evaluated that a low molecular weight polysaccharide (LMW-ABP) isolated from *Agaricus blazei* Murill, which inhibits the adhesion of human colon cancer cells HT-29 by suppressing the expression level of e-selectin protein and gene. In addition, LMW-ABP also inhibited NF-κB expression and nuclear translocation [31].

Another research group suggested that modified apple polysaccharides (MAP) suppressed the migration and invasion of colorectal cancer cells (HT-29 and SW620) induced by lipopolysaccharide. MAP significantly decreased LPS-induced expression of TLR4, cyclooxygenase 2, matrix metallopeptidase 9 (MMP9), matrix metallopeptidase 2 (MMP-2), inducible nitric oxide synthase, and prostaglandin E2, and increased the protein expression of the inhibitor of κBα and NF-κB p65 in cytoplasm when it was given in combination with LPS. These results showed that MAP possessed clinical value in preventing CRC cell metastasis [32].

P53 Apoptosis Pathway

P53, a tumor suppressor, plays a key role in cellular stress and tumor suppression, including DNA repair, cell cycle arrest, vascular growth inhibition and cell apoptosis [33]. Recent studies found that polysaccharide-induced apoptosis of cancer cells was dependent on the existence of functional p53. Foreign scholar Park et al. demonstrated the role of p53-rugulated tumor-suppressing pathways in promoting the anticancer effects of fucoidan. The results indicated that fucoidan inhibited cell viability, induced apoptosis and DNA damage in two p53 isogenic HCT116 (p53+/+ and p53-/-) cell lines. Thus, fucoidan could be a novel therapeutic option for CRC treatment regardless of the p53 status [34]. SFPSA, isolated from the rhizomes of *Stachys flordana* Schuttl ex Benth, composed of rhamnose, glucuronic acid, galacturonic acid, glucose, galactose and arabinose in a molar ratio of 7.75:1.65:14.92:1.87:33.17:40.64 and with an average molecular weight of 168 kDa. Their results showed that SFPSA could suppress the growth and proliferation of HT-29 cells in a time- and concentration-dependent manner for 48 h, and induce the apoptosis and augment the accumulation of G_2/M phase. In addition, SFPSA could increase the activity of caspase-3 and the mRNA expression level of p53 and Bax, and down-regulate Bcl-2 mRNA expression level. Indicating that SFPSA-induced apoptosis of HT-29 cells might be via regulation of apoptosis-associated p53 gene expressions [35].

Jiang et al. reported that *Ganoderma lucidum* polysaccharides (GLPs), extracted from spores, mycelia and fruiting bodies of *Ganoderma lucidum*, possess anti-cancer activities. These results suggested that GLPs could reactivate mutant p53 in colorectal cancer HT29 ($p53^{R273H}$) and SW480 ($p53^{R273H\&P309S}$) cells while applied alone or together with 5-fluorouracil (5-FU) to inhibit cell growth and induce cell apoptosis. Therefore, targeting mutant p53 with GLPs combined other chemotherapeutics may be a novel treatment strategy for colon cancer [36].

Another research evaluated the molecular changes involved in p53 pathway in HT-29 cells treated with fermented bean (cv. Bayo Madero) polysaccharide extract with human gut flora for 24 h by PCR array. Their results showed that 72 of 84 human p53-mediated signal transduction response genes involved in apoptosis, cell proliferation and cell cycle presented significant expression changes, providing insight about the mechanism underlying its overall chemoprotective function against colon carcinogenesis [37].

MAPK Signaling Pathway

The mitogen-activated protein kinases (MAPKs), a kind of intracellular serine/threonine protein kinase, transfer the extracellular stimulus signal into the intracellular to affect tumor cells, including cell death and apoptosis [38]. Liang et al. reported that *Ganoderma lucidum* polysaccharide (GLP) induced cell death/apoptosis on HCT-116 cells in a time- and dose-dependent manner. GLP increased the Bax/Bcl-2-ratio through mitochondrial-mediated caspase-dependent intrinsic pathway to induce apoptosis in HCT-116 cells. Furthermore, GLP-induced apoptosis is related to the MAPK signaling pathway and cell cycle arrest at S phase [39]. Another research group found that *Ganoderma atrum* polysaccharide (PSG-1) possessed anti-tumor activity *in vivo* and *in vitro*. PSG-1 inhibited the proliferation of CT26 cells through the activation of peritoneal macrophages in co-culture system. Furthermore, PSG-1 increased TLR4 and NF-κB expression, IκBα degradation and p38 MAPK phosphorylation to induce CT26 cell apoptosis [40].

Cell Cycle

The cell cycle is defined as the whole process of continuous mitotic cells from the end of one mitosis to the end of the next mitosis, and divided into four phases, including G1 phase, S phase, G2 phase and M phase [41]. Cell cycle is accurately regulated by intracellular genetic material. Disturbance of the cell cycle in eukaryotic cells at any point will block the whole process of cell replication [42]. Therefore, cell cycle arrest will be a potential target in antitumor treatment. Studies have shown that polysaccharides could induce cell cycle arrest to inhibit the proliferation of tumor cells. *Salvia miltiorrhiza* Bunge polysaccharides (SMP), extracted by water boiling and ethanol precipitation with high purity, composed of Gal, Glc, and GalUA with the mole percentages of 64.5%, 31.1%, and 4.4%. Wang et al.

demonstrated that SMP could arrest the cell cycle at S phase and increase the production of the intracellular reactive oxygen species to induce LoVo cells apoptosiss [43]. PS and CS, isolated from *Salicornia herbacea*, showed the anti-proliferation effect on HT-29 cell line in a dose-dependent fashion. Furthermore, PS and CS induced G2/M arrest and increased the expression of p53 gene and p21 gene to suppress the growth of HT-29 cells [44].

Foreign scholars Park et al. studied that fucoidan decreased the cell viability and induced apoptosis in HCT-116 cells. Further analysis showed that fucoidan resulted in G1 arrest in the cell cycle progression, including the upregulation of cyclin-dependent kinase (CDK) inhibitors expression, such as p21WAF1/CIP1 and p27KIP1 [34]. American scholars Yun et al. also demonstrated that fucoidan treatment significantly suppressed the growth and induced apoptosis in HT-29 colon cancer cells. Fucoidan reduced cyclin (cyclin D1 and cyclin E) and cyclin-dependent kinase (CDK2 and CDK4) expression, which causes cell cycle arrest. In addition, fucoidan upregulated the ratio of Bax/Bcl-2, and the expression of cleaved caspase-3 and cleaved PARP1 protein [45].

A water-soluble polysaccharide (PAP), extracted from the fruiting bodies of *Pleurotus abalonus*, consisted of Man, Rib, Rha, GluA, Glu and Gal with the mole percentages of 3.4%, 1.1%, 1.9%, 1.4%, 87.9% and 4.4%. PAP was shown to exert a dose-dependent anti-proliferative effect against LoVo cancer cells through inducing cell-cycle arrest at the S phase. They also found that PAP could increase intracellular ROS production which was a key mediator in PAP-induced cell growth inhibition [46]. Mao et al. investigated that the effects of Wolfberry polysaccharide on the proliferation and apoptosis of SW480 and Caco-2 human colon cancer cells. Their results showed that LBP could inhibit the growth and clone formation of SW480 and Caco-2 cells, and decrease cyclin (cyclin D and cyclin E) and CDK2 protein expression, leading to the cell cycle arrest at G0/G1 phase [47]. *Orostachys japonicas* polysaccharide (OJPI) resulted in a marked increase of cells in the G0 (sub G1) and G2/M phases to induce apoptosis in HT-29 cells [48] and safflower polysaccharide also induced the cell cycle arrest of HT-29 cells [49]. In addition, SHPSA, obtained from *Sargassum horneri*, could also suppress the growth of human colon cancer DLD cells in a dose-dependent manner through inducing the cell cycle arrest at G2/M phase [50].

P1, isolated from *Phellinus linteus*, effectively inhibited the size and weight of tumor in HT-29 tumor-bearing mice. It also increased the weight of mice and has no toxicity to mammals. Furthermore, P1 induced S cell cycle arrest in a dose-dependent manner in HT-29 cells [51].

PI3K/AKT Signaling

PI3K/AKT signaling pathway is closely related to cell differentiation, growth, apoptosis and movement, and if the PI3K/AKT signaling pathway is activated, the proliferation of tumor cells will be uncontrolled [52]. Studies have shown that polysaccharides exert anti-tumor activities by inhibiting PI3K/AKT signaling pathway [53]. Sun et al. reported that a water-soluble polysaccharide SPS2p, isolated from the whole grass of *Scutellaria barbata*, composed of arabinose, mannose, glucose and galactose at the ratio of 1.31:1.00:3.59:1.59, and the molecular weight of SPS2p is 2.6×10^4 Da. Their results showed that SPS2p could inhibit the proliferation, induce the apoptosis and block the EMT process of human colon cancer HT29 cells. SPS2p also down-regulated the ratio of p-AKT/AKT in HT-29 cells, indicating that the PI3K/AKT signaling pathway was blocked, which may be related to the apoptosis [54].

Foreign scholar Han et al. studies the anti-proliferation and anti-migration effects of fucoidan on human colon cancer HT29 cells. Fucoidan downregulated the PI3K-AKT-mTOR signaling pathway, increased the expression of cleaved caspase-3 and decreased cancer sphere formation [53].

Other Apoptotic Pathways

Cell apoptosis is strictly controlled by genes that independently control orderly cell death, and defined as the maintenance of cellular homeostasis. When the regulation of apoptosis is uncontrolled, the cells will be excessive proliferation or apoptosis, which caused the occurrence of diseases such as cancer [55]. In recent years, in addition to the regulation of polysaccharides on apoptosis mechanisms mentioned above, other apoptotic pathways have been discovered.

Liu et al. reported that Tea polysaccharide (TPS) effectively prevented AOM/DSS-induced CRC, and they studied the possible mechanisms. They found that TPS decreased the tumor incidence, tumor size, and significantly suppressed the infiltration of pro-inflammatory cells and the secretion of pro-inflammatory cytokines IL-6 via balancing the cellular microenvironment. In addition, TPS inhibited the activation of STAT3 and regulated the expression of downstream genes including MMP2, cyclin D1, survivin, and VEGF *in vitro* and *in vivo* to exert anti-tumor effects [56].

The Wnt/β-catenin signaling pathway is associated with the development of cancers, and involved in various intracellular biological processes. Abnormal activation in genes of the Wnt/β-catenin signaling pathway is observed early in the development of colon cancers. Several studies shown that polysaccharides can prevent the development of colon cancer by regulating the Wnt/β-catenin signaling pathway. Foreign scholars Song et al. investigated the anti-tumor activity of PL against human colon cancer SW480 cells *in vitro* and *in vivo*. Their results showed that PL significantly reduced the expression of β-catenin, cyclin D1, and T-cell factor/lymphocyte enhancer binding factor (TCF/LEF) transcription activity *in vitro*. In addition, PL inhibited the tumor growth of SW480 cells implanted into nude mice, and decreased β-catenin expression. This study showed that PL suppresses tumor growth, invasion, and angiogenesis via inhibiting the Wnt/β-catenin signaling in SW480 cells [57].

Tumor metastasis is a multiple cascade process that involves tumor cell adhesion, invasion, migration, angiogenesis, distant metastasis sites, and tumor cell proliferation [58]. Many studies shown that polysaccharides possess anti-metastasis activity against tumor cells. A low molecular weight polysaccharide (LMW-ABP), extracted from the fruiting bodies of *Agaricus blazei* Murill, could significantly suppress the interaction between E-selectin and sialyl Lewis X (sLe^x) and the adhesion of HT-29 cells to human umbilical vein endothelial cells (HUVECs) in dose-dependent fashion in static conditions, and down-regulate the gene and protein expression of α-1,3-fucosyltransferase-VII (FucT-VII) and sLe^x. These results indicated that LMW-ABP could inhibit the metastasis of colon cancer cells via blocking the interaction between E-selectin and sLe^x [31].

EFFECTS OF POLYSACCHARIDES ON THE GUT MICROFLORA

Several studies have shown that DSS-induced colitis could significantly alter the gut microbiota in mice, and polysaccharides greatly altered the structure of gut microbiota, induced bacteria to produce short-chain fatty acids to maintain a proper intestinal pH, maintained the integrity of a structurally and functionally intact gastrointestinal tract, and promoted the maturation of immune cells and the apoptosis of colon cancer cells [59, 60]. *Ganoderma lucidum* polysaccharide (GLPs) possesses the mitigative effect on AOM/DSS-induced colon cancer (CRC) via gut microbiota. Their results showed that GLPs treatment significantly decreased the relative abundance

(RA) of cecal *Oscillospira*, along with an unknown genus of *Desulfovibrionaceae*, and down-regulated 7 genes related to the reduction of lipolysis in adipocytes, among which Acca1b, Fabp4, Mgll and Scd1 were associated with cancer. These results suggested that the effect of GLPs on colon cancer was related to the decrease of specific bacteria and the regulation of tumor-related genes [61].

A previous study demonstrated the inhibitory effects of a polysaccharide isolated from the Traditional Chinese Medicine (TCM) – Licorice on CT-26 tumor-bearing mouse model. GCP markedly altered the gut microbiota between the model group and GCP group, and significantly reduced the relative abundance of Enterorhabdus, Odoribacter, Ruminiclostridiu_5, Ruminococcac-eae_UCG_010 and Lachnospirac-eae_UCG_001. Furthermore, fecal transplantation experiments showed that transplanting the feces of GCP-treated mice, to a certain extent, could inhibit tumor growth and metastasis. These results indicated that GCP possesses anti-tumor effects via influencing the gut microbiota composition [62]. Another research showed the chemopreventive effect of polysaccharides from common beans (*Phaseolus vulgaris* L.) on AOM-induced colon cancer. PE could produce short-chain fatty acids (SCFA), such as acetate, propionate and butyrate, in the large intestine. In addition, PE reduced the number of aberrant crypt foci (ACF) and increased the expression of Bax and caspase-3 to induce cell apoptosis. These data showed that PE decreased ACF, affected the expression of apoptotic genes, and altered the concentration of butyrate [63].

ABOUT OUR RESEARCH

Rhizopus nigricans, a zygomycete filamentous fungus belonging to the order Mucorales, is widely used in brewing and pharmaceutical industry due to its functions of biocatalysis and biotransformation [64]. Our previously reported that exopolysaccharide (EPS1-1), isolated from

Rhizopus nigricans, consisted of glucose, mannose, galactose and fructose in the molar ratio of 5.89:3.64:3.20:1.00 with weight average molecular weight of 9.7×10^3 g/mol. *In vitro* experiments showed that EPS1-1 could markedly suppress the proliferation of human colorectal carcinoma HCT-116 cells and induce apoptosis via cell cycle arrest at S phase. EPS1-1 resulted in dissipation of mitochondrial membrane potential, accumulation of reactive oxygen species (ROS), up-regulation of Bax and p53 expression and down-regulation of Bcl-2 expression in transcription level, which indicated that EPS1-1-induced apoptosis also through mitochondrial pathway [65].

Cao, Hou et al. demonstrated the anti-tumor and immune activities of EPS1-1 in S180 bearing mice. The results revealed that EPS1-1 significantly inhibited the proliferation of S180 cells and increased the proliferation ability of spleen lymphocytes. In comparison with the control groups, EPS1-1 consumption remarkably declined the weights of tumor and the inhibition rates. Notably, the prophylactic treatment of EPS1-1 could more efficiently suppressed the growth of S180 tumor than direct administration of EPS1-1. Meanwhile, EPS1-1 could prolong the survival of S180 tumor bearing mice. The results suggested that the mechanism of anti-tumor effect of EPS1-1 may be mediated by increased immune activity in host [66].

Yu, Kong et al. evaluated the immune-enhancing activities of EPS1-1 *in vitro* and *in vivo*. Results suggested that EPS1-1 stimulated the proliferation of lymphocyte and enhanced the activities of macrophages by increasing the activities of phagocytosis and acid phosphatase, the generation of NO and the gene expression levels of IL-2, TNF-α and iNOS. EPS1-1 could remarkably promote the immunity of immunosuppressed and normal mice via the increase of loaded swimming time, footpad swelling, organ index and the secretion of IL-2 and TNF-α in serum, suggesting that EPS1-1 boosts the body immunity through humoral immunity and cellular immunity [67].

Yu, Sun et al. reported that EPS1-1 possesses the anti-metastasis effects against mouse colon cancer CT26 cells *in vitro* and *in vivo*. Results showed that EPS1-1 inhibited the migration, invasion and adhesion abilities, and the enzyme activity and expression levels of matrix metalloproteinases (MMPs) in dose-dependent fashion in CT26 cells. In addition, similar results were obtained in lung metastasis mice. EPS1-1 decreased the expression of vascular endothelial growth factor (VEGF), microvessel density (MVD), and vimentin to inhibit angiogenesis in lung tissue, which suggesting that EPS1-1 could inhibit metastasis by suppressing invasion and angiogenesis *in vitro* and *in vivo* [68].

Song et al. investigated the inhibitory effect of EPS1-1 on AOM/DSS-induced colitis-associated colorectal cancer (CAC) in mice. EPS1-1 effectively relieved pathological symptoms, including weight loss, piloerection, hematochezia and insensitivity caused by AOM/DSS. Compared with the model group, EPS1-1 significantly down-regulated the expression levels of COX-2, β-catenin, Cyclin D1, C-Myc, Ki-67 and PCNA protein, and Bcl-2 gene, while up-regulated the expression of p53 and Bax gene. Furthermore, EPS1-1 notably reduced the number of cells positive for CD68, F4/80 and NF-κB, and decreased the concentrations of inflammatory factors, such as TNF-α and IL-6 in serum. These data indicated that EPS1-1 possesses the chemopreventive effect on CAC [69].

Another research tested the beneficial effects of EPS1-1 on the intestinal immunity of AOM/DSS-induced colorectal cancer mice. EPS1-1 could resist hydrolysis in an artificial stomach. Compared with the model group, EPS1-1 altered gut microbiota and increased the concentration of total SCFAs in the feces of colorectal cancer mice. Importantly, EPS1-1 also increased the villus length, ratio of villus length and crypt depth in colonic tissues, and promoted the number of acid mucus-secreting goblet cells in mice. These observations revealed that EPS1-1 may play a vital role in the improvement of intestinal function in colorectal cancer mice [68].

Taking all of these results into account, EPS1-1 has strong potential as efficient bio-secure anti-colon cancer drug or adjuvant drug in clinical applications.

CONCLUSION

Polysaccharides, which possesses various biological activities and has not been reported to be toxic to normal cells, is internationally known as "tumor biological response regulator" and has obtained extensive attention. So far, the research, development and application of polysaccharides have made great progress. We have summarized a variety of active polysaccharides to the colon cancer prevention and the inhibition function, which shows remarkable effects. The biological properties of polysaccharides correlate closely with their chemical structures, especially their monosaccharide compositions, molecular weights, types of glycosidic linkages, and positions of glucosidic linkages.

Therefore, future studies should further explore the relationships between the biological properties of polysaccharides and their chemical structures. In addition, the biological activities of polysaccharides mainly present the cells *in vitro* and the corresponding reflected in animal models, while these effects were different from the actual function of the human body. In the further studies, the efficacy of polysaccharides should be applied to the clinical to confirm the anti-cancer activities, which provides the theoretical basis for their potential role in the prevention and treatment of colon cancer, and lays a foundation for the future research and development of medicine fields.

REFERENCES

[1] Xiao long, J, Qiang, P & Min, W (2018). Anti-colon-cancer effects of polysaccharides, A mini-review of the mechanisms. *International Journal of Biological Macromolecules*, *114*, 1127-1133.

[2] Safa, T J, Ons, Z, Efstathia, I, Ichrak, RC, Meriam, H, Vassilios, R, Riadh, K & Khadija, EB (2017), Mertensene, a Halogenated Monoterpene, Induces G2/M Cell Cycle Arrest and Caspase Dependent Apoptosis of Human Colon Adenocarcinoma HT29 Cell Line through the Modulation of ERK-1/-2, AKT and NF-kappaB Signaling. *Marine Drugs*, *15*.

[3] Wei, D, Lan Wei, Z, Hua Xi, Y, Xue, H, Ying Chun, Z & Liang, X (2018). Exopolysaccharides produced by Lactobacillus strains suppress HT-29 cell growth via induction of G0/G1 cell cycle arrest and apoptosis. *Oncology Letters*, *16*, 3577-3586.

[4] Venkataraman, D, Sharavan, R, Reham Mohammed, B, Sureshbabu Ram, P, Shiva, DS, Hariharan, N & Krishnan, S (2015). *In vitro* evaluation of anticancer properties of exopolysaccharides from Lactobacillus acidophilus in colon cancer cell lines. *In Vitro Cell Dev Biol Anim*, *52*, 163-173.

[5] S, O, KA, J, JD, B & FM, G (1997). Hereditary nonpolyposis colorectal cancer. *Annals of Oncology* 8, 1151-1156.

[6] Fang, Z, Jun Jun, S, Kiran, T, Fei, H, Jian Guo, Z & Zhao Jun, W (2017). Anti-Cancerous Potential of Polysaccharide Fractions Extracted from Peony Seed Dreg on Various Human Cancer Cell Lines Via Cell Cycle Arrest and Apoptosis. *Frontiers Pharmacology*, *8*, 102.

[7] Panida, S, Stefani, L, Kyungchul, C, Ita Novita, S, Hyog Young, K & Yun Kyung, L (2018). Toll-Like Receptor 2-Mediated Suppression of Colorectal Cancer Pathogenesis by Polysaccharide A From Bacteroides fragilis. *Frontiers Microbiology*, *9*, 1588.

[8] Kyung Soo, N & Yun Hee, S (2008). Chemopreventive effects of polysaccharides extract from Asterina pectinifera on HT-29 human colon adenocarcinoma cells. *BMB reports*, 277-280.

[9] Yan, L, Lei, X, Yun Zhe, C, Ge, S, Jun, H, Guo Dong, W, Peng Ying, Z & Kao Shan, C (2019). Structural characteristics and anticancer/antioxidant activities of a novel polysaccharide from Trichoderma kanganensis." *Carbohydrate polymers*, 205, 63-71.

[10] Juan Juan, P, Zhen Bin, W, Hai Le, M & Jing Kun, Y (2015). Structural features and antitumor activity of a novel polysaccharide from alkaline extract of Phellinus linteus mycelia. *Carbohydrate polymers*, 115, 472-477.

[11] Gang, Z, Ying, J, Huan, S, Ning Xin, Z & Li, H (2013). Immunopontentiating activities of the purified polysaccharide from evening primrose in H22 tumor-bearing mice. *Int J Biol Macromol*, 52, 280-285.

[12] Tamara, B, Nancy, PC, Matía, VE, Betty, M & Elisa, AZ (2011). Antioxidant capacity of sulfated polysaccharides from seaweeds. A kinetic approach. *Food Hydrocolloids*, 25, 529-535.

[13] Ye, Y, Fang Yuan, G, Xing Xin, W, Yang, S, Yi Hua, L, Ting, C & Qiang, X (2008). Anti-inflammatory and immune-suppressive effect of flavones isolated from Artemisia vestita. *Journal of Ethnopharmacology*, 120, 1-6.

[14] Ya Feng, Z, Shuai, Z, Qi, W, Xu, L, Liang Mei, L, Yu Ting, T, Jian Bo, X & Bao Dong, Z (2016). Characterization and hypoglycemic activity of a beta-pyran polysaccharides from bamboo shoot (Leleba oldhami Nakal) shells. *Carbohydrate polymers*, 144, 438-446.

[15] Dao Yuan, R, Ning, W, Jian Jun, G, Li, Y & Xing Bin, Y (2016). Chemical characterization of Pleurotus eryngii polysaccharide and its tumor-inhibitory effects against human hepatoblastoma HepG-2 cells. *Carbohydrate polymers*, 138, 123-133.

[16] Ming, S, Wen Yan, Z, Qing Peng, X, Yun Hong, Z & Bin, W (2015). Lentinan reduces tumor progression by enhancing

gemcitabine chemotherapy in urothelial bladder cancer. *Surgical Oncology*, *24*, 28-34.

[17] Hai Rong, C, Shan Shan, L, Yu Ying, F, Xiao Ge, G, Miao, H, Jia, W, Xiao Yan, Z, Gui Hua, T & Yi Fa, Z (2011). Comparative studies of the antiproliferative effects of ginseng polysaccharides on HT-29 human colon cancer cells. *Med Oncol*, *28*, 175-181.

[18] Yuki, M, Koichi, I, Morichika, K & Hiroaki, N (2010). A polysaccharide extracted from Grifola frondosa enhances the anti-tumor activity of bone marrow-derived dendritic cell-based immunotherapy against murine colon cancer. *Cancer Immunol Immunother*, *59*, 1531-1541.

[19] Daniel, RL, Olaia, MI, Catalina Fernandez de Ana, P, Arturo, RB, Manuel, VA, Andrea, DD, Alba, C, Cecilia, P & Angélica, F (2019). *In Vitro* Anti-proliferative and Anti-invasive Effect of Polysaccharide-rich Extracts from Trametes Versicolor and Grifola Frondosa in Colon Cancer Cells. *International Journal of Medical Sciences*, *16*, 231-240.

[20] Can Hong, W, Shu Xian, Y, Li, GLW & Li Li C (2018). Carboxymethyl pachyman (CMP) reduces intestinal mucositis and regulates the intestinal microflora in 5-fluorouracil-treated CT26 tumour-bearing mice. *Food Funct*, *9*, 2695-2704.

[21] Sanjeev, G, George, K, Eva, S & Bertrand, J (2009). The mitochondrial death pathway: a promising therapeutic target in diseases, *Journal of Cellular and Molecular Medicine.*, *13*, 1004-1033.

[22] Zhi Qiang, Q, Ying Wan, W, Ye Li, L, Yi Qi, L, Ling, Z & Dan Li, Y (2017). Icariin prevents hypertension-induced cardiomyocyte apoptosis through the mitochondrial apoptotic pathway. *Biomedicine & Pharmacotherapy*, *88*, 823-831.

[23] Hua Yi, S, Jia Le, S, Ya Lin, Z, Zhen Hu, L, Ruo Kun, Y, Kai, Z, Jie, X & Xin, Z (2014). Induction of apoptosis in HCT-116 colon cancer cells by polysaccharide of Larimichthys crocea swim bladder. *Oncol Lett*, *9*, 972-978.

[24] Yu Jin, K, Jin Woo, J, Yung Hyun, C & Chung Ho, R (2013). Soy soluble polysaccharide induces apoptosis in HCT116 human colon cancer cells via reactive oxygen species generation. *Mol Med Rep*, 8, 1767-1772.

[25] Ana, AFP, Laura, CB, Guadalupe, GA, Ramón, GGG, Minerva, RG, Rosalía, RC, Jorge, AAG & Guadalupe, LP (2008). Composition and Chemopreventive Effect of Polysaccharides from Common Beans (Phaseolus vulgaris L.) on Azoxymethane-Induced Colon Cancer. *J. Agric. Food Chem*, 56, 8737-8744.

[26] Jing Lin, W, Wei Yong, L, Xiao, H, Ying, L, Qiang, L, Zi Ming, Z & Kai Ping, W (2017). A polysaccharide from Lentinus edodes inhibits human colon cancer cell proliferation and suppresses tumor growth in athymic nude mice. *Oncotarget*, 8, 610-623.

[27] Zeng Enni, L, You Jin, Y, Yu Tong, G, Ren Cai, W, Qiu Long, H & Xing Yao, X (2015). Inhibition of migration and induction of apoptosis in LoVo human colon cancer cells by polysaccharides from Ganoderma lucidum. *Mol Med Rep*, 12, 7629-7636.

[28] Ki Mun, K & Jin-Hyun, A (2015). Differential Regulation of NF-κB Signaling during Human Cytomegalovirus Infection. *Journal of Bacteriology and Virology*, 45, 159.

[29] Dai, C, Xin Yu, Z, Meng, M, Li Rong, H, Cai Jiao, L, Li Hua, H, Wen Tao, Q & Chun Ling, W (2016). Inhibitory effect on HT-29 colon cancer cells of a water-soluble polysaccharide obtained from highland barley. *Int J Biol Macromol*, 92, 88-95.

[30] Jun, L, Ya Hong, Z, Zhi Qiang, T, Fang, L, Ying, S, Yao, L & Pei Yuan, X. (2017). Astragalus polysaccharides protect against dextran sulfate sodium-induced colitis by inhibiting NF-kappacapital VE, Cyrillic activation. *Int J Biol Macromol*, 98, 723-729.

[31] Ji Cheng, L, Li Ling, Y, Chun, Z, Li, F, Li, Z, Yu, L, Ying Cai, N, Xue Yan, L, Xian Chun, W & Yong Xu, S (2010). A polysaccharide isolated from Agaricus blazei Murill inhibits sialyl Lewis X/E-selectin-mediated metastatic potential in HT-29 cells

through down-regulating α-1,3-fucosyltransferase-VII (FucT-VII). *Carbohydrate polymers*, *79*, 921-926.

[32] Dian, Z, Yu Hua, L, Man, M, Feng Liang, J, Zheng Gang, Y, Yang, S Lei, F, Jin, M, Xin, Z, Li, L & Qi Bing, M (2013). Modified apple polysaccharides suppress the migration and invasion of colorectal cancer cells induced by lipopolysaccharide. *Nutr Res*, *33*, 839-848.

[33] Katerina, A, He, Y, Bhupinder, B, Maurizia, G & Eleftherios, PD (2000). p53 Gene Mutation, Tumor p53 Protein Overexpression, and Serum p53 Autoantibody Generation in Patients with Breast Cancer. *Clinical Biochemistry*, *33*, 53-62.

[34] Hye Young, P, Shin-Hyung, P, Jin-Woo, J, Dahye, Y, Min Ho, H, Dae-Sung, L, Grace, C, Mi-Jin, Y, Jeong Min, L, Do-Hyung, K, Gi-Young, K, Il-Whan, C, Suhkmann, K, Heui-Soo, K, Hee-Jae, C & Yung Hyun, C (2017). Induction of p53-Independent Apoptosis and G1 Cell Cycle Arrest by Fucoidan in HCT116 Human Colorectal Carcinoma Cells. *Mar Drugs*, *15*, 154.

[35] Li Ping, M, Cui Li, Q, Ming Chun, W, Dan, G, Lin, C, Hong, Y & Xiao Xiong, Z (2013). Preparation, preliminary characterization and inhibitory effect on human colon cancer HT-29 cells of an acidic polysaccharide fraction from Stachys floridana Schuttl. ex Benth. *Food Chem Toxicol*, *60*, 269-276.

[36] Dan, J, Ling Yao, W, Tong, Z, Zhao Yu, Z, Ren Xia, Z, Jing Ji, J, Yong, C & Fei, Wa (2017). Restoration of the tumor-suppressor function to mutant p53 by Ganoderma lucidum polysaccharides in colorectal cancer cells. *Oncol Rep*, *37*, 594-600.

[37] R, CV, RG, GG, BL, GO, B, DO & G, LP. (2010). Bean (Phaseolus vulgaris L.) polysaccharides modulate gene expression in human colon cancer cells (HT-29). *Food Research International*, *43*, 1057-1064.

[38] Eva Marina, S, Sebastian, L, Cristina, B, Christian, S, Stefan, K, Helmut, B, Heiko, H, Andreas, J, Thomas, K & David, H (2018). Targeting tumor cell plasticity by combined inhibition of NOTCH

and MAPK signaling in colon cancer. *The Journal of Experimental Medicine*, *215*, 1693-1708.

[39] Zen Gen Ni, L, You Jin, Y, Yu Tong, G, Ren Cai, W, Qiu Long, H & Xing Yao, X (2014). Chemical characterization and antitumor activities of polysaccharide extracted from Ganoderma lucidum. *Int J Mol Sci*, *15*, 9103-9116.

[40] Shen Shen, Z, Shao Ping, N, Dan Fei, H, Wen Juan, L & Ming Yong, X (2013). Immunomodulatory effect of Ganoderma atrum polysaccharide on CT26 tumor-bearing mice. *Food Chem*, *136*, 1213-1219.

[41] Hideaki, M, Yoshito, N, Nobuya, I, Akinori, S & Kunio, K (2009). A signature-based method for indexing cell cycle phase distribution from microarray profiles. *BMC Genomics*, *10*, 137.

[42] Yan, W, Zhi, C, Min, W, Yan Ling, J, Ai Jun, Y & Min, L (2018). COPB2 suppresses cell proliferation and induces cell cycle arrest in human colon cancer by regulating cell cycle-related proteins. *Exp Ther Med*, *15*, 777-784.

[43] Xing Yu, W, An Ning, G, Ya Dong, J, Yan, Z & Xing Bin, Y (2018). Antitumor effect and molecular mechanism of antioxidant polysaccharides from Salvia miltiorrhiza Bunge in human colorectal carcinoma LoVo cells. *Int J Biol Macromol*, *108*, 625-634.

[44] Ryu, DS, Seon-Hee, K & Dong-Seok, L (2009). Anti-Proliferative Effect of Polysaccharides from Salicornia herbacea on Induction of G2/M Arrest and Apoptosis in Human Colon Cancer Cells. *J. Microbiol. Biotechnol*, *19*, 1482-1489.

[45] Chul Won, Y, Seungpil, Y, Jun Hee, L, Yong Seok, H, Yeo Min, Y, Daniel, A & Sang Hun, L (2016). Silencing Prion Protein in HT29 Human Colorectal Cancer Cells Enhances Anticancer Response to Fucoidan. *Anticancer Res*, *36*, 4449-4458.

[46] Dao Yuan, R, Ya Dong, J, Xing Bin, Y, Li, Y, Jian Jun, G & Yan, Z (2015). Antioxidant and antitumor effects of polysaccharides

from the fungus Pleurotus abalonus. *Chem Biol Interact*, *237*, 166-174.

[47] Fang, M, Bing Xin, X, Zhen, J, Jun Wei, Z, Xia, H & Jun Ming, G (2011). Anticancer effect of Lycium barbarum polysaccharides on colon cancer cells involves G0/G1 phase arrest. *Med Oncol*, *28*, 121-126.

[48] Deok-Seon, R, Geum-Ok, B, Eun-Young, K, Ki-Hoom, K & Dong-Seok, L (2010). Effects of polysaccharides derived from Orostachys japonicus on induction of cell cycle arrest and apoptotic cell death in human colon cancer cells. *BMB Rep*, *43*, 750-755.

[49] Liang, A, Jiang Hong, Z, Tai Jun, Z, Xiao Qing, L, Qiong, Z & Jun, C (2017). Analysis of the inhibitory effect of safflower polysaccharide on HT29 colorectal cancer cell proliferation and its relevant mechanism. *Biomedical Research*, *28*, 2966-2970.

[50] Ping, S, Jia, L, Xiao Xiao, C, Zhong Xiang, F & Pei Long, S (2015). Structural features and antitumor activity of a purified polysaccharide extracted from Sargassum horneri. *Int J Biol Macromol*, *73*, 124-130.

[51] Shi, Z, Dong Feng, J, You Gui, L, Tian Bao, L, Zhi Qiang, L & Hua Ping, C (2013). Activation of P27kip1-cyclin D1/E-CDK2 pathway by polysaccharide from Phellinus linteus leads to S-phase arrest in HT-29 cells. *Chem Biol Interact*, *206*, 222-229.

[52] Chuang, Y, Ming Huan, W, Jun De, Z & Qiang, C (2017). Upregulation of miR-542-3p inhibits the growth and invasion of human colon cancer cells through PI3K/AKT/survivin signaling. *Oncol Rep*, *38*, 3545-3553.

[53] Yong-Seok, H, Jun Hee, L & Sang Hun, L (2015). Fucoidan inhibits the migration and proliferation of HT-29 human colon cancer cells via the phosphoinositide-3 kinase/Akt/mechanistic target of rapamycin pathways. *Mol Med Rep*, *12*, 3446-3452.

[54] Peng Da, S, Dong, S & Xu Dong, W (2017). Effects of Scutellaria barbata polysaccharide on the proliferation, apoptosis and EMT of

human colon cancer HT29 Cells. *Carbohydrate polymers*, *167*, 90-96.

[55] Paul, GE (1997). Apoptosis, haemopoiesis and leukaemogenesis. *Baittikre's Clinical Haematology*, *10*, 561-576.

[56] Li Qiao, L, Shao Ping, N, Ming Yue, S, Jie Lun, H, Qiang, Y, De Ming, G & Ming Yong, X (2018). Tea Polysaccharides Inhibit Colitis-Associated Colorectal Cancer via Interleukin-6/STAT3 Pathway. *J Agric Food Chem*, *66*, 4384-4393.

[57] Kyoung-Sub, S, Ge, L, Jong-Seok, K, Kai Peng, J, Tae-Dong, K, Jin-Pyo, K, Seung-Bo, S, Jae-Kuk, Y, Hae-Duck, P, Byung-Doo, H, Kyu, L & Wan-Hee, Y (2011). Protein-bound polysaccharide from Phellinus linteus inhibits tumor growth, invasion, and angiogenesis and alters Wnt/b-catenin in SW480 human colon cancer cells. *BMC Cancer*, *11*, 307.

[58] Myoung-Sook, S, Su-Hyun, H, Taek-Joon, Y, Sung-Han, K & Kwang-Soon, S (2017). Polysaccharides from ginseng leaves inhibit tumor metastasis via macrophage and NK cell activation. *Int J Biol Macromol*, *103*, 1327-1333.

[59] Xiao Jun, H, Shao Ping, N & Ming Yong, X (2017). Interaction between gut immunity and polysaccharides. *Critical Reviews in Food Science and Nutrition*, *57*, 2943-2955.

[60] Min, L, Bao Hong, W, Meng Hui, Z, Mattias, R, Sheng Yue, W, Hao Kui, Z, Yan, Z, Jian, S, Xiao Yan, P, Mei Ling, Z, Hua, W, Yu, C, Hai Feng, L, Jian, Z, Ming Ming, S, Yun Ping, Q, Wei, J, Chao Ni, X, Leon, MS, Sheng Li, Y, Elaine, H, Hui Ru, T, Guo Ping, Z, Jeremy, KN, Lan Juan, L & Li Ping, Z (2007). Symbiotic gut microbes modulate human metabolic phenotypes. *Proceedings of the National Academy of Sciences*, *105*, 2117-2122.

[61] Jian Ming, L, Cheng, Z, Rong, L, Li Juan, G, Shi, Yi, O, Liu, L & Xi Chun, P (2018). Ganoderma lucidum polysaccharide alleviating colorectal cancer by alteration of special gut bacteria and regulation of gene expression of colonic epithelial cells. *Journal of Functional Foods*, *47*, 127-135.

[62] Xiao, Yu Z, Shu Wu, Z, Xin Bo, S, Jian Wei, J, Zha Yi, Z, Hui Fang, Z, Hui, F, Huan Tian, C, Shuo, H, Min Jie, F, Xiao Min, L & Yu Hong, B (2018). Inhibition effect of glycyrrhiza polysaccharide (GCP) on tumor growth through regulation of the gut microbiota composition. *J Pharmacol Sci*, *137*, 324-332.

[63] Ana, AFP, Laura, CB, Guadalupe, GA, Ramón, GGG, Minerva, RG, Rosalía, RC, Jorge, AAG & Guadalupe, LP (2008). Composition and chemopreventive effect of polysaccharides from common beans (Phaseolus vulgaris L.) on azoxymethane-induced colon cancer. *J Agric Food Chem*, *56*, 8737-8744.

[64] Zhi Hong, W, Guo Chuang, C, Peng Ying, Z, Lei, Z, Li Nan, Z & Kao Shan, C (2018). Rhizopus nigricans polysaccharide activated macrophages and suppressed tumor growth in CT26 tumor-bearing mice. *Carbohydrate polymers*, *198*, 302-312.

[65] Wen Qian, Y, Guo Chuang, C, Peng Ying, Z & Kao Shan, C. (2016). Purification, partial characterization and antitumor effect of an exopolysaccharide from Rhizopus nigricans. *Int J Biol Macromol*, *82*, 299-307.

[66] Jian Feng, C, Dong, H, Jing Bo, L, Lei, Z, Peng Ying, Z, Nan, Z & Kao Shan, C (2016). Anti-tumor activity of exopolysaccharide from Rhizopus nigricans Ehrenb on S180 tumor-bearing mice. *Bioorg Med Chem Lett*, *26*, 2098-2104.

[67] Zhi Dan, Y, Meng, Li K, Peng Ying, Z, Qing Jie, S & Kao Shan, C (2016). Immune-enhancing activity of extracellular polysaccharides isolated from Rhizopus nigricans. *Carbohydrate polymers*, *148*, 318-325.

[68] Zhi Dan, Y, Qing, Jie S, Jing, L, Xiu Juan, Z, Ge S, Guo Dong, W, Peng, Ying Z & Kao Shan, C (2018). Polysaccharide from Rhizopus nigricans inhibits the invasion and metastasis of colorectal cancer. *Biomed Pharmacother*, *103*, 738-745.

[69] Ge, S, Yan, L, Zhi Dan, Y, Lei, X, Jing, L, Kao Shan, C & Peng, Ying, Z (2019). The inhibitory effect of polysaccharide from

Rhizopus nigricans on colitis-associated colorectal cancer. *Biomed Pharmacother*, *112*, 108593.

In: Colorectal Cancer
Editor: Masayoshi Yamaguchi

ISBN: 978-1-53616-598-2
© 2020 Nova Science Publishers, Inc.

Chapter 2

THE ROLE OF REGUCALCIN AS A SUPPRESSOR IN HUMAN COLORECTAL CANCER

*Masayoshi Yamaguchi**, *PhD*
Cancer Biology Program, University of Hawaii Cancer Center,
University of Hawaii at Manoa, Honolulu, HI, US

ABSTRACT

Regucalcin plays a crucial role as a regulator of transcription signaling activity, and its lowered expression or activity may contribute in the promotion of human carcinogenesis. Higher regucalcin expression in the tumor tissues has been demonstrated to prolong survival of patients with cancer of various types, including pancreatic cancer, breast cancer, liver cancer, and lung adenocarcinoma. The involvement of regucalcin in human colorectal cancer was investigated in the current study. The regucalcin gene expression and survival data of 62 patients were obtained though the Gene Expression Omnibus (GEO) database (GSE12945), to analysis outcome. Data of gene expression showed that prolonged survival in colorectal cancer patients is associated with higher regucalcin

---

* Corresponding Author's E-mail: yamamasa11555@yahoo.co.jp.

gene expression in tumor tissues. Overexpression of regucalcin depressed colony formation, proliferation and death of human colorectal carcinoma RKO cells *in vitro*. Mechanistically, overexpressed regucalcin induced G1 and G2/M phase cell cycle arrest of RKO cells through suppression of multiple signaling pathways including Ras, Akt, MAP kinase and SAPK/JNK. Interestingly, overexpressed regucalcin caused elevation of the tumor suppressers p53 and Rb, and cell cycle inhibitor p21. Moreover, c-*fos*, c-jun, NF-κB p65, β-catenin, and Stat3, transcription factor, were repressed by overexpressed regucalcin. This study suggests that regucalcin plays a crucial role as a suppressor in human colorectal cancer, and that the suppressed regucalcin gene expression may predispose patients to the promotion of colorectal cancer. Overexpressed regucalcin with the gene delivery may play a role as a novel therapy of colorectal cancer.

Keywords: colorectal cancer, regucalcin, RKO cell, colony formation, cell proliferation, cell death

INTRODUCTION

Regucalcin was originally discovered as a kind of calcium-binding protein [1]. The regucalcin gene (*rgn*) is localized on the X chromosome [2-4]. This protein was found to have reversible effects on the activity of various calcium-regulated enzymes [5, 6], suggesting a role as the novel inhibitory protein of calcium signaling in cell regulation [6]. Moreover, regucalcin has been demonstrated to play a pivotal role as a suppressor of manifold signaling pathways and its linked to transcription activity in various types of cells [7, 8]; this protein plays a regulatory role in the inhibition of various signaling pathways implicated in calcium homeostasis, various protein kinases and protein phosphatases, repression of cytosolic protein synthesis, nuclear DNA and RNA synthesis, and regulation of nuclear gene expression [9]. Moreover, regucalcin has been found to suppress the proliferation [10] and apoptotic cell death mediated through diverse signaling molecules in the cells of various types of tissues [11]. Thus, regucalcin may play a pivotal role in maintaining cell homeostasis [12].

Notably, the expression of regucalcin has been shown to be lowered in the tumor tissues of mammalian and human subjects *in vivo* [13, 14], suggesting that diminished regucalcin gene expression may induce the promotion of carcinogenesis [13, 14]. We demonstrated that survival was prolonged in patients of pancreatic cancer [15], breast cancer [16], hepatocellular carcinoma [17], and lung cancer [18]] with the higher regucalcin expression in their tumor tissues as compared with those of lower regucalcin expression. With supporting of these findings, overexpressed regucalcin was shown to exhibit repressive effects on the growth of human pancreatic cancer MIA PaCa-2 cells [15], MDA-MB 231 breast cancer cells [16], liver cancer HepG2 cells [17], and lung adenocarcinoma A549 cells [18] *in vitro*. Regucalcin may play a potential role as a suppressor in the development of carcinogenesis of human subjects, demonstrating its significance as a novel biomarker in the diagnosis of human cancer.

Adenocarcinoma is the predominant malignancy found in the colon and rectum [19]. Colorectal cancer is the third most common cancer diagnosed in the developed world [20, 21]. The average 5-year survival rate remains poor at 55% [22], although the development of new drugs has improved the survival rate of colorectal cancer patients. The prognosis of colorectal cancer remains poor in spite of the development of novel therapeutic strategies [22-25]. Human colorectal cancer represents a heterogenous group of diseases, and its molecular classification is increasingly important [22-25]. Characterization of novel biomarker targets may lead to prolong the survival of colorectal cancer. Biomarkers may have a potential role in screening, diagnosis, progonosis and monitoring disease [22-25]. Mutations in the *KRAS* gene in ~ 40% of tumors have been reported to be induced by genetic and epigenetic alterations [26-28].

The involvement of regucalcin in human colorectal cancer was not been investigated. We were undertaken to determine whether or not regucalcin is involved in the suppression of human colrorectal cancer. Notably, we found that prolonged survival of colorectal cancer patients is associated with higher regucalcin gene expression in the tumor tissues as evaluated by the analysis of gene expression using the Gene Expression Omnibus (GEO) database (GSE17891) [29]. In addition, overexpressed regucalcin was shown to inhibit the growth of human colorectal cancer RKO cells *in vitro*. Our findings support the view that the diminished regucalcin gene expression predisposes patients with colorectal cancer, suggesting a new strategy as a therapeutic tool with the gene therapy in human cancer.

INVOLVEMENT OF REGUCALCIN IN COLORECTAL CANCER PATIENTS

An involvement of regucalcin in the patients of human colorectal cancer has been investigated [29]. We analyzed the expression levels of regucalcin in colorectal tumor tissues of human subjects *in vivo*. We compared the regucalcin gene expression in the tumor tissues of the colorectal cancer patients. Regucalcin gene expression and survival data of 62 patients of colorectal cancer were obtained though the Gene Expression Omnibus (GEO) database (GSE12945) for outcome analysis [29]. These datasets contained gene expression data derived from the Affymetrix U133A array. Microarray analysis was performed as previously described [15-18]. Expression and raw expression data (CEL files) were summarized and normalized using the Robust Multi-array Average algorithm and the Bioconductor package affy (http://www.bioconductor.org/packages/2.0/bioc/html/affy.html).

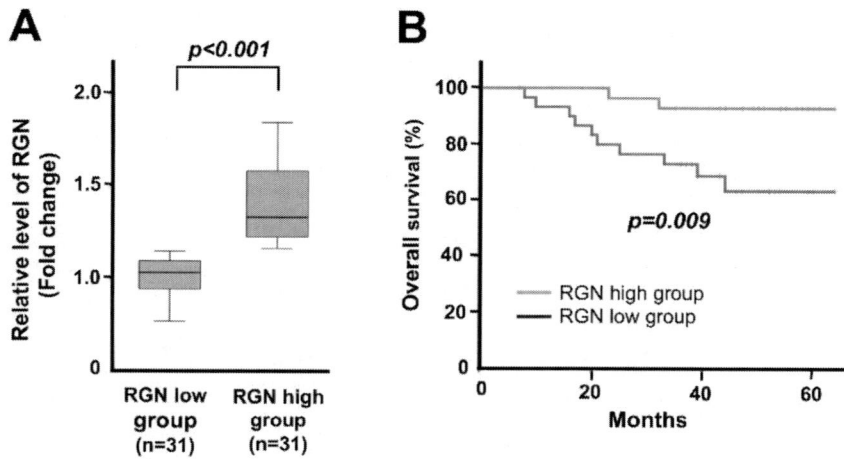

Figure 1. Decreased regucalcin gene expression is correlated with poor outcome of patients with colorectal cancer. A: The group of patients is separated into 2 groups (high and low of regucalcin gene expression). High group of the regucalcin gene expression showed a statistically significant difference as compared with that of low group. B: Kaplan-Meier curve indicated that survival curves for colorectal cancer patients were significantly prolonged in high group of the regucalcin gene expression as compared with that of low expression. Abbreviations: RGN; regucalcin. Figure was cited from Ref. 29.

Colorectal cancer patients were classified into two groups with high (31 patients) or low (31 patients) of regucalcin mRNA expression in the colorectal tumor tissues. As the group of patients with higher regucalcin mRNA expression was compared to the group of patients with lower regucalcin mRNA expression, a significant difference was found in two groups. Analysis of Kaplan-Meier curve showed that survival of the group with higher regucalcin mRNA expression in the tumor tissues of colorectal patients is predominantly prolonged as compared with that of the group with lower regucalcin mRNA expression (Figure 1). This finding supported the view that suppressed regucalcin gene expression may contribute in the promotion or aggressiveness of carcinogenesis in human colorectal cancer. Downregulated regucalcin gene expression may lead to a worse clinical outcome of cancer patient.

OVEREXOPRESSED REGUCALCIN SUPPRESSES COLONY FORMATION OF HUMAN COLORECTAL CANCER CELLS

Moreover, to elucidate a translational mechanism for this clinical finding, we used epithelial RKO cells originated from male adult patients of colorectal carcinoma, which were obtained from the American Type Culture Collection [29]. RKO cells were suitable as a transfection host. RKO cells were cultured in the Dulbecco's Modification of Eagle's Medium (DMEM; with 4.5 g/L glucose, L-glutamine and sodium pyruvate) containing fetal bovine serum (FBS) and antibiotics (100 μg/mL penicillin and 100 μg/mL streptomycin; P/S). RKO wild-type cells were transfected with pCXN2 vector expressing cDNA encoding human full length (900 bp) regucalcin (regucalcin cDNA/pCXN2) [30]. To assay transient transfection, RKO cells were grown on 24-well plates in reaching on subconfluence. Regucalcin cDNA/pCXN2 and empty pCXN2 vector alone were transfected into RKO cells using the synthetic cationic lipid components, a Lipofectamine reagent [30]. After incubation for overnight, Geneticin (600 μg/ml) was added to culture wells, and cells were cultured to select transfected cells for 3 weeks. After that, cells were plated at limiting dilution to isolate transfectants. Survival clones were isolated, transferred to 35-mm dishes, and grown in the medium without Geneticin. We obtained clone 1 and 2 of transfectants with stable expression of regucalcin, and regucalcin levels in these clones were increased by 7.4- or 10.9-fold as compared with that of wild-type cells respectively. Clone 2 was used in the following experiment.

Then, clone 2 was used to determine the effects of overexpressed regucalcin on the growth of RKO cells *in vitro*. RKO wild-type cells or transfectants were seeded into 6-well dishes at a density of 1×10^3/well and cultured in medium containing 10% FBS and 1% P/S under the condition of 5% CO_2 and 37°C for 7 days, when visible clonies were formed on the plates [31]. The obtained colonies were washed with

PBS and fixed with methanol (0.5 ml per well) for 20 min at room temperature, and then washed 3 times with PBS. Finally, colonies were stained with 0.5% crystal violet for 30 min at room temperature. Stained cells were washed 4 times with PBS. The plates were air-dried for 2 hours at room temperature. The colonies containing more than 50 cells were counted under a microscope. Overexpressed regucalcin was showed to suppress colony formation of RKO cells without inducing direct cell toxicity with necrotic or apoptotic cell deaths *in vitro* [29]. This study demonstrates a crucial role of regucalcin as a suppressor in the growth of human colorectal cancer cells. Endogenous regucalcin may play a suppressive role in the development of human colorectal cancer.

OVEREXPRESSED REGUCALCIN SUPPRESSES THE PROLIFERATION OF HUMAN COLORECTAL CANCER CELLS

Moreover, we investigated whether overexpressed regucalcin exhibits the suppressive effects on cell proliferation and it is attenuated in the presence of various inhibitors related to the proliferation *in vitro* [29]. RKO wild-type cells (1×10^5/ml per well) or ROK cells (1×10^5/ml per well) transfected with regucalcin cDNA were cultured in DMEM containing 10% FBS and 1% P/S using a 24-well plate for 1, 2, 3, 4 or 7 days in a water-saturated atmosphere containing 5% CO_2 and 95% air at 37°C [29]. In separate experiments, RKO wild-type cells or transfectants were cultured in DMEM containing 10% FBS and 1% P/S in the presence of either sodium butyrate (10 and 100 µM), roscovitine (10 and 100 nM), sulphoraphan (1 and 10 nM), dibucaine (0.1 or 1 µM), Bay K 8644 (0.1 or 1 µM), PD98059 (1 or 10 µM), wortmannin (0.1 or 1 µM), 5, 6-dichloro-1-β-D-ribofuranosylbenzimidazole (DRB; 0.1 or 1 µM), or gemcitabine (50 or 100 nM) for 3 days. After culture, cell number in suspended medium was counted as described in the following. To detach cells on each well, culture dishes were incubated for 2 min at 37°C after the addition of the solution (0.1 ml per well) of 0.05% trypsin plus EDTA in Ca^{2+}/Mg^{2+}-free PBS, and then cells were detached through pipetting after the addition of DMEM (0.9 ml) containing 10% FBS and 1% P/S [29, 30]. Medium containing the suspended cell (0.1 ml) was mixed by adding 0.1 ml of 0.5% trypan blue staining solution. The number of cells with viability were counted under a microscope using a Hemocytometer plate using cell counter. For each dish, we took the average of two counting. Cell number was showed as number per well of plate. Wild-type cells were cultured for 3 days in the presence of butyrate (10 and 100 μM) [31], roscovitine (10 and 100 nM) [32] or sulforaphane (1 and 10 nM) [33]. Proliferation of wild-type cells was repressed in the presence of these inhibitors [29]. Effects of these inhibitors were not potentiated in transfectants (Figure 3B). This result suggested that overexpressed regucalcin induces G1 and G2/M phase cell cycle arrest in RKO cells, although further experiments are remained to confirm using immunofluorescence assay.

Next, we determined an involvement of signaling factors in the exhibition of suppressive effects of overexpressed regucalcin on cell proliferation [29]. Proliferation of RKO wild-type cells was repressed by dibucaine (0.1 or 1 μM), an inhibitor of calcium/calmodulin-dependent protein kinases [35], and staurosporine (10 or 100 nM), a calcium signaling protein kinase C-related inhibitor [36], and PD98059 (1 or 10 μM), an inhibitor of extracellular signal-regulated kinas (ERK) and mitogen-activated protein kinase (MAPK) [37]. Blocking of these pathways did not potentiate suppressive effects of overexpressed regucalcin on cell proliferation.

Wortmannin (0.1 or 1 μM) is an inhibitor of phosphatidylinositol 3-kinase (PI3K) [38]. DRB is an inhibitor of transcriptional activity with RNA polymerase II inhibition [39]. Gemcitabine is a strong antitumor agent that induces nuclear DNA damage [40]. These inhibitors caused a repression of the proliferation of wild-type cells (Figure 4C). Such effects were not potentiated in transfectants. These results suggest that overexpressed regucalcin suppresses various signaling processes linked to cell proliferation, and that regucalcin-overexpressing cells lead to the lack of responses for above inhibitors.

As described above, the mechanistic characterization in exhibiting depressive effects of overexpressed regucalcin on the proliferation of RKO cells was investigated using various inhibitors that regulate cell-signaling pathways. Exhibiting repressive effects of overexpressed regucalcin on the proliferation of RKO cells were not potentiated in the presence of butyrate, roscovitine or sulphoraphan that induce cell-cycle arrest. Butyrate induces an inhibition of G1 progression [32]. Roscovitine is a potent and selective inhibitor of the cyclin-dependent kinase cdc2, cdk2m and cdk5 [33]. Sulforaphane induces G2/M phase cell cycle arrest [34]. Overexpressed regucalcin was suggested to cause G1 and G2/M phase cell cycle arrest in RKO cells. Such findings were shown in various types of cells, including normal rat kidney proximal tubular epithelial NRK52E cells [41], rat hepatoma H4-II-E cells [31], and human cancer cells of various types [15-18] *in vitro*. Importantly, overexpressed regucalcin reduced expression of p21, a cell cycle inhibitor, supporting the view that regucalcin plays a role in cell cycle arrest [15-18].

SUPPRESSIVE EFFECTS OF OVEREXPRESSED REGUCALCIN ON THE PROLIFERATION ARE INDEPENDENT ON CELL DEATH

The effects of overexpressed regucalcin on the death of RKO cells were investigated [29]. RKO wild-type cells (1×10^5/ml per well) cells or RKO cells (1×10^5/ml per well) transfected with regucalcin cDNA were cultured in DMEM containing 10% FBS and 1% P/S using a 24-

wells plate for 3 days on reaching subconfluency, and then were cultured for additional 24 hours in the presence or absence of either Bay K 8644 (0.1 or 1 µM), tumor necrosis factor-α (TNF-α; 0.1 or 1 ng/ml) or lipopolysaccharoide (LPS; 0.1 or 1 µg/ml) [40]. In separate experiments, RKO wild-type cells (1×10^5/ml per well) or transfectants were cultured for 3 days in reaching on subconfluence, and then were cultured for an additional 24 hours in the presence or absence of either Bay K 8644 (1 µM), TNF-α (1 ng/ml) or LPS (1 µg/ml), which induces apoptotic cell death [42], with or without caspase-3 inhibitor (10 µM) for 24 hours [31]. After culture, cells were detached by the addition of sterilized solution (0.1 ml per well) of 0.05% trypsine plus EDTA in Ca^{2+}/Mg^{2+}-free PBS into each well as described in the section of cell proliferation assay, and then cell number was countered. The number of wild-type cells was decreased by culture with Bay K 8644, TNF-α, or LPS]. Overexpression of regucalcin did not lead to the death of wild-type cells, and apoptotic cell death-inducing factors did not cause the cell death of transfectants. This result suggests that the revelation of repressive effects of overexpressed regucalcin on the proliferation of RKO cells are not resulted from causing of cell death.

Moreover, we investigated whether the effects of overexpressed regucalcin on cell death are mediated through caspase-3. RKO wild-type cells and transfectants in reaching on subconfluence were cultured in the presence of Bay K 8644 (1 µM), TNF-α (1 ng/ml) or LPS (1 µg/ml) with or without caspase-3 inhibitors (10 µM) for 24 hours [29]. The effects of LPS or TNF-α on cell death were not revealed in the presence of caspase-3 inhibitor. The stimulatory effects of Bay K 8644, TNF-α or LPS on cell death was not exhibited in transfectants cultured with or without caspase-3 inhibitor. Thus, regucalcin was suggested to prevent cell death by decreasing the activity of caspase-3 that activates DNA fragmentation in the nucleus, leading to apoptotic cell death. Thus, the exhibition of suppressive effects of overexpressed regucalcin on the proliferation of RKO cells were not resulted from cell death.

OVEREXPRESSED REGUCALCIN REGULATES EXPRESSION OF PROTEINS LINKED TO CELL SIGNALING AND TRANSCRIPTION ACTIVITY

Mechanistically, we investigated whether overexpressed regucalcin regulates the expression of key proteins, which are implicated to signaling pathways and transcription activity, using Western blot analysis [29]. RKO wild-type cells, control vector cDNA-transfected cells, or regucalcin cDNA-transfected cells were plated in 100 mm dishes at a density of 1×10^6 cells/well in 10 ml of DMEM containing 10% FBS and 1% P/S, and they were cultured for 3 days. After culture, cells were washed three times with cold PBS and removed from the dish by scraping using cell lysis buffer with the addition of the inhibitors of protease and protein phosphatase. The lysates were then centrifuged at 12,000 rpm, at 4°C for 10 min. The protein concentration of the supernatant obtained was determined for Western blotting using the Bio-Rad Protein Assay Dye with bovine serum albumin as a standard. Then, the supernatant was stored at -80°C until used. Samples of 40 micrograms of supernatant protein per lane were separated by SDS polyacrylamide gel electrophoresis (12%, SDS-PAGE) and transferred to nylon membranes for immunoblotting using specific antibodies against various proteins, which were obtained from Cell Signaling Technology and Santa Cruz Biotechnology, Inc. Rabbit anti-regucalcin antibody was obtained from Abcam. Target protein was incubated with one of the primary antibodies (1:1000) including phosphorylated type of various proteins for overnight at 4°C, and followed by horseradish peroxidase-conjugated secondary antibodies (diluted 1:2000). The immune reactive blots were visualized with a SuperSignal West Pico Chemiluminescent Substrate detection system according to the manufacture's instruction. β-Actin (diluted 1:2000) was used as a loading control. Three blots from independent experiments were scanned on an Epson Perfection 1660 Photo scanner, and bands quantified using Image J.

Overexpressed regucalcin was found to decrease the levels of Ras, Akt, phosphor-Akt, MAPK, phosphor-MAPK, SAPK/JNK, phosphor-SAPK/JNK, and PI3 kinase 100α [29]. These results suggest that overexpressed regucalcin suppresses activation of Ras-linked signaling pathways in RKO cells. Interestingly, overexpression of regucalcin elevated protein levels of p53 and Rb, tumor suppressors, and p21, an inhibitor of cell cycle [29]. In addition, overexpressed regucalcin diminished c-fos, c-jun, NF-κB p65, β-catenin, Stat3, and phospho-stat3 which are transcription factors linked to cell proliferation in RKO cells [29]. Thus, we found the change in protein levels (14 molecules), which may be major signaling proteins related to the proliferation of cancer cell. However, other various proteins are implicated in the proliferation of cancer cell. Further investigation is needed to determine involvement of other proteins.

As mentioned previously, the suppressive effects of overexpressed regucalcin on the proliferation of RKO cells were not potentiated in the presence of dibucaine, an inhibitor of calcium/calmodulin-dependent protein kinases, staurosporine, an inhibitor of protein kinase C, wortmannin, an inhibitor of PI3/Akt signaling pathway, and PD98059, an inhibitor of ERK/MAP kinase-related to signaling pathway [29]. Overexpressed regucalcin was shown to reveal depressive effects on the proliferation due to inhibiting various signaling pathways, which are implicated to Ca^{2+}-dependent kinases, PI3/Akt, and ERK/MAPK in RKO cells. Thus, regucalcin was potential as a suppressor in diverse signaling pathways in human cancer cells [29]. Furthermore, results with Western blot analysis showed that overexpressed regucalcin leaded to decrease in various proteins that participate signal pathways linked to Ras, Akt, MAPK, SAPK/JNK, and PI3 kinase in RKO cells [29]. The exhibition of suppressive effects of regucalcin, which is mediated through regulation of various signaling pathways, were also observed in various types of human cancer cells, including pancreatic MIA-PaCa2 cells [15], MDA-MB-231 human breast cancer cells [16], human liver cancer HepG2 cells [17], and human lung cancer A549 cells [18] *in vitro*.

OVEREXPRESSED REGUCALCIN REGULATES GENE EXPRESSION

The suppressive effects of overexpressed regucalcin on the proliferation of RKO cells were not altered by culture with DRB, an inhibitor of transcriptional activity with RNA polymerase II inhibition [39]. The suppressive effects of overexpressed regucalcin on the proliferation of RKO cells were not potentiated by culture with gemcitabine, which is used in the therapy of human cancer as an antitumor agent that induces DNA damage in the nuclei [40]. Gemcitabine inhibits the proliferation and stimulates apoptotic cell death in various types of cancer cells [40]. Our result suggests that regucalcin partly regulates pathways implicated to the mode of action of gemcitabine. Regucalcin has been demonstrated to directly suppress DNA and RNA synthesis using isolated rat liver nuclei [43].

Notably, regucalcin has been shown to play a role in the regulation of cell nuclear function [9]. Importantly, overexpressed regucalcin has been demonstrated to enhance the gene expressions of *p53* and *Rb,* a suppressor of tumor, and p21, an inhibitor of cell cycle, and suppress the gene expressions of *ras*, c-*jun* and c-*myc*, an oncogene, due to binding to nuclear DNA in cloned rat hepatoma H4-II-E cells *in vitro* [9, 43]. Moreover, overexpressed regucalcin was found to elevate the protein levels of *p53*, *Rb* and p21 and diminish that of ras, c-fos, c-fos, NF-κB p65, β-catenin and Stat3, which are transcription factors linked to cancer cell proliferation, in RKO cells *in vitro*. These findings may support the view that endogenous regucalcin plays a pivotal role to mediate depressive effects on the growth of cancer cells due to regulating the expression of various proteins linked to transcription factors, tumor suppressors and oncogenes linked to tumor development. Regucalcin binds to DNA [43] and regulates the gene expressions of various proteins in the nucleus of normal and cancer cells [9, 43].

REGUCALCIN MAY INHIBIT METASTASIS OF CANCER CELLS

Overexpressed regucalcin was shown to prevent colony formation of RKO cells *in vitro* [29]. Such effects of overexpressed regucalcin on colony formation in RKO cells may be resulted from the proliferation suppressed by overexpression of regucalcin. Colorectal cancer cells may express a particularly aggressive metastatic phenotype of primary neoplastic cells to regional lymph nodes, liver, adrenal glands, contralateral lung, brain, and bone marrow [19, 22]. Overexpression of regucalcin may lead to suppression of colony formation and metastasis of colorectal cancer.

CONCLUSION

Prolonged survival is demonstrated to be associated with higher regucalcin gene expression in the tumor tissues of colorectal cancer patients, and that overexpressed regucalcin represses the proliferation of human colorectal cancer RKO cells *in vitro*. Endogenous regucalcin with higher expression plays a potential role as a suppressor in the development of human colorectal cancer, and that downregulated regucalcin leads to progression of carcinogenesis. Previously, we showed that survival is prolonged in the patients of pancreatic cancer [15], breast cancer [16], hepatocellular carcinoma [17], and lung adenocarcinoma [18] with higher regucalcin expression in the tumor tissues, and that overexpressed regucalcin suppresses growth of their related human cancer cells *in vitro* [15-18]. Thus, regucalcin is proposed to play a crucial role as a suppressor of carcinogenesis in various types of human cancer. Downregulated regucalcin gene expression may predispose patients to promotion of human cancer. Delivery of the regucalcin gene, which is overexpressed in tumor tissues, may provide a new strategy as a therapeutic tool for human cancer.

REFERENCES

[1] Yamaguchi M, Yamamoto T (1978) Purification of calcium binding substance from soluble fraction of normal rat liver. *Chem Pharm Bull* (Tokyo) 26: 1915-1918.

[2] Shimokawa N, Yamaguchi M (1993) Molecular cloning and sequencing of the cDNA coding for a calcium-binding protein regucalcin from rat liver. *FEBS Lett* 327: 251-255.

[3] Shimokawa N, Matsuda Y, Yamaguchi M (1995) Genomic cloning and chromosomal assignment of rat regucalcin gene. *Mol Cell Biochem* 151:157-163.

[4] Thiselton DL, McDowall J, Brandau O, Ramser J, d'Esposito F, Bhattacharga SS, Ross MT, Hardcastle AJ, Meindl M (2002) An integrated, functionally annotated gene map of the DXS8026-ELK1 internal on human Xp11.3-Xp11.23: Potential hotspot for neurogenetic disorders. *Genomics* 79:560-572.

[5] Yamaguchi M, Mori S (1988) Effect of Ca^{2+} and Zn^{2+} on 5'-nucleotidase activity in rat liver plasma membranes: Hepatic calcium-binding protein (regucalcin) reverses the Ca^{2+} effect. *Chem Pharm Bull* (Tokyo) 36: 321-325.

[6] Yamaguchi M (2000) Role of regucalcin in calcium signaling. *Life Sci* 66: 1769-1780.

[7] Yamaguchi M (2005) Role of regucalcin in maintaining cell homeostasis and function. *Int J Mol Med* 15:372-389.

[8] Yamaguchi M (2011) Regucalcin and cell regulation: role as a suppressor in cell signaling. *Mol Cell Biochem* 353:101-137.

[9] Yamaguchi M (2013) Role of regucalcin in cell nuclear regulation: Involvement as a transcription factor. *Cell Tissue Re*s 354: 331-341.

[10] Yamaguchi M (2013) Suppressive role of regucalcin in liver cell proliferation: Involvement in carcinogenesis. *Cell Prolif* 46: 243-253.

[11] Yamaguchi M (2013) The anti-apoptotic effect of regucalcin is mediated through multisignaling pathways. A*poptosis* 18:1145–1153.

[12] Yamaguchi M (2017) In: The Role of Regucalcin in Cell Homeostasis and Disorder. Nova Science Publishers, Inc., New York, USA.

[13] Yamaguchi M (2015) Involvement of regucalcin as a suppressor protein in carcinogenesis. Insight into the gene therapy. *J Cancer Res Clin Oncol* 141:1333-1341.

[14] Murata T, Yamaguchi M (2014) Alternatively spliced variants of the regucalcin gene in various human normal and tumor tissues. *Int J Mol Med* 34:1141-1146.

[15] Yamaguchi M, Osuka S, Weitzmann MN, El-Rayes BF, Shoji S, Murata T Prolonged survival in pancreatic cancer patients with increased regucalcin gene expression: Overexpression of regucalcin suppresses the proliferation in human pancreatic cancer MIA PaCa-2 cells *in vitro*. *Int J Oncol* 48:1955-1964.

[16] Yamaguchi M, Osuka S, Weitzmann MN, Shoji S, Murata T (2016) Increased regucalcin gene expression extends survival in breast cancer patients: overexpression of regucalcin suppresses the proliferation and metastatic bone activity in MDA-MB-231 human breast cancer cells *in vitro*. *Int J Oncol* 49:812-822.

[17] Yamaguchi M, Osuka S, Weitzmann MN, Shoji S, Murata T (2016) Prolonged survival in hepatocarcinoma patients with increased regucalcin gene expression: HepG2 cell proliferation is suppressed by overexpression of regucalcin *in vitro*. *Int J Oncol* 49:1686-1694.

[18] Yamaguchi M, Osuka S, Shoji S, Weitzmann MN, Murata T (2017) Survival of lung cancer patients is prolonged with higher regucalcin gene expression: suppressed proliferation of lung adenocarcinoma A549 cells in vitro. *Mol Cell Biochem* 430:37–46.

[19] Porter MG, Stoeger SM (2017) A typical colorectal neoplasms. *Surg Clin N Am* 97:641-656.

[20] American Cancer Society. Cancer facts & figures 2016. Atlanta (GA): American Cancer Society; 2016.

[21] Siegel RI, Miller KD, Jemal A (2016) Cancer statics, *CA Cancer J Clin* 66:7-30.

[22] Brenner H, Kloor M, Pox CP (2014) Colorectal cancer. *Lancet* 383:1490-1502.

[23] Alnabulsi A, Murray GI (2016) Integrative analysis of the colorectal cancer proteome; potential clinical impact. *Expert Rev Proteomics* 13:917-927.

[24] Alnabulsi A, Swan R, Cash B, Alnabulsi A, Murray GI (2017) The differential expression of omega-3 and omega-6 fatty acid metabolizing enzymes in colorectal cancer and its prognostic significance. *Brit J Cancer* 116:1612-1620.

[25] Carini F, Mazzola M, Rappa F, Jurjus A, Geagea AG, Kattar A AL, Bou-Assi T, Jurius R, Damiani P, Leone A, Tomasello G (2017) Colorectal carcinogenesis: Role of oxidative stress and antioxidants. *Anticancer Research* 37:4759-4766.

[26] Colussi D, Brandi G, Bazzoli F, Ricciardiello L (2013) Molecular pathways involved in colorectal cancer: implications for disease behavior and prevention. *Int J Mol Sci* 14: 16365–16385.

[27] Kudryavtseva AV, Lipatova AV, Zaretsky AR, Moskalev AA, Fedorova MS, Rasskazova AS, Shibukhova GA, Snezhkina AV, Kaprin AD, Alekseev BY, Dmitriev AA, Krasnov GS (2016) Important molecular genetic markers of colorectal cancer. *Oncotarget* 7: 53959–53983.

[28] Jones RP, Sutton PA, Evans JP, Clifford R, McAvoy A, Lewis J, Rousseau A, Mountford R, McWhirter D, Malik HZ (2017) Specific mutations in KRAS codon 12 are associated with worse overall survival in patients with advanced and recurrent colorectal cancer. *Brit J Cancer* 116:923-929.

[29] Yamaguchi M, Osuka S, Murata T (2018) Prolonged survival of colorectal cancer patients is associated with higher regucalcin gene expression: Overexpressed regucalcin suppresses growth of human colorectal carcinoma cells *in vitro*. *Int J Oncol* 53:1313-1322.

[30] Staub E, Groene J, Heinze M, Mennerich D, Roepcke S, Klaman I, Hinzmann B, Castanos-Velez E, Pilarsky C, Mann B, Brummendorf T, Weber B, Buhr HJ, Rosenthal A (2009) An expression module of WIPF1-coexpressed genes identifies patients with favorable prognosis in three tumor types. *J Mol Med* (Berl) 87:633-644.

[31] Misawa H, Inagaki S, Yamaguchi M (2002) Suppression of cell proliferation and deoxyribonucleic acid synthesis in cloned rat hepatoma H4-II-E cells overexpressing regucalcin. *J Cell Biochem* 84: 143-149.

[32] Charollais RH, Buquet C, Mester J (1990) Butyrate blocks the accumulation of cdc2 mRNA in late G1 phase but inhibits both early and late G1 progression in chemically transformed mouse fibroblasts BP-A31. *J Cell Physiol* 145:46-52.

[33] Meijer L, Borgne A, Mulner O, Chong JP, Blow JJ, Inagaki N, Inagaki M, Deleros JG, Moulinoux JP (1997) Biochemical and cellular effects of roscovitine, a potent and selective inhibitor of

the cyclin-dependent kinases cdc2, cdk2 and cdk5. *Eur J Biochem* 243:527-536.

[34] Singh SV, Herman-Antosiewice A, Singh AV, Lew KL, Strivastava SK, Kamath R, Brown KD, Zhang L, Baskaran R (2004) Sulforaphan-induced G2/M phase cell cycle arrest involves checkpoint kinase 2-mediated phosphorylation of cell division cycle 25C. *J Biol Chem* 279:25813-25822.

[35] Yamaguchi M, Daimon Y (2005) Overexpression of regucalcin suppresses cell proliferation in cloned rat hepatoma H4-II-E cells: Involvement of intracellular signaling factors and cell cycle-related genes. *J Cell Biochem* 95: 1169-1177.

[36] Tamaoki T, Nomoto H, Takahashi I, Kato Y, Morimoto M, Tomita E (1986) Staurosporine, a potent inhibitor of phospholipid/Ca^{2+} dependent protein kinase. *Biochem Biophys Res Commun* 135: 397-402.

[37] Serrano-Nascimento C, da Silva Teixeira S, Nicola JP, Nachbar RT, Masini-Repiso AM, Nunes MT (2014) The acute inhibitory effect of iodide excess on sodium/iodide symporter expression and activity involves the PI3K/Akt signaling pathway. *Endocrinology* 155:1145-1156.

[38] Peleck SL, Charest DL, Mordret GP, Siow YL, Palaty C, Campbell D, Chaslton L, Samiei M, Sanghera JS (1993) Networking with mitogen-activated protein kinases. *Mol Cell Biochem* 127: 157-169.

[39] Palangat M, Grass JA, Langelier MF, Coulombe B, Landick R (2011) The RPB2 flap loop of human RNA polymerase II is dispensable for transcription initiation and elongation. *Mol Cell Biol* 31:3312-3325.

[40] Tang SC, Chen YC (2014) Novel therapeutic targets for pancreatic cancer. *World J Gastroenterol* 20:10825-10844.

[41] Nakagawa T, Sawada N, Yamaguchi M (2005) Overexpression of regucalcin suppresses cell proliferation of cloned normal rat

kidney proximal tubular epithelial NRK52E cells. *Int J Mol Med* 16: 637-643.

[42] Izumi T, Yamaguchi M (2004) Overexpression of regucalcin suppresses cell death in cloned rat hepatoma H4-II-E cells induced by tumor necrosis factor-α or thapsigargin. *J Cell Biochem* 92: 296-306.

[43] Tsurusaki Y, Yamaguchi M (2004) Role of regucalcin in liver nuclear function: Binding of regucalcin to nuclear protein or DNA and modulation of tumor-related gene expression. *Int J Mol Med* 14: 277-281.

In: Colorectal Cancer ISBN: 978-1-53616-598-2
Editor: Masayoshi Yamaguchi © 2020 Nova Science Publishers, Inc.

Chapter 3

AN ARYL HYDROCARBON RECEPTOR AGONIST SUPPRESSES THE GROWTH OF HUMAN COLORECTAL CANCER CELLS

Masayoshi Yamaguchi*, PhD
Cancer Biology Program, University of Hawaii Cancer Center,
University of Hawaii at Manoa, Honolulu, HI, US

ABSTRACT

Human colorectal cancer, which represents a heterogenous group of diseases, is the third most common cancer with the average 5-year survival rate at 55%. Characterization of novel biomarker targets with molecular classification may lead to prolonging survival of colorectal cancer. The aryl hydrocarbon receptor (AHR) is transcriptionally active in the form of a heterodimer with the AHR nuclear translocator, which then binds to the xenobiotic responsive element. AHR was initially discovered via its ligand, the polychlorinated hydrocarbon, 2, 3, 7, 8-tetrachlorodibenzo-*p*-dioxin (TCDD). We investigated whether TCDD, an agonist of AHR signaling, regulates the growth of RKO human colorectal cancer cells *in vitro*. Treatment with TCDD (0.1-100 nM)

---

* Corresponding Author's E-mail: yamamasa11555@yahoo.co.jp.

revealed suppressive effects on colony formation and proliferation of RKO cells, and stimulated death of these cells with subconfluence. These effects of TCDD were abolished by pretreatment with CH223191, an inhibitor of AHR signaling. Western blot analysis showed that TCDD treatment decreased AHR levels and elevated CYP1A1 levels, indicating a stimulation of AHR signaling. TCDD treatment caused the increase in NF-κB p65 and β-catenin, although it did not have an effect on Ras levels. Importantly, TCDD treatment increased the levels of p53, Rb, p21, and regucalcin, which are suppressors of the growth of tumor cells. Of note, effects of TCDD on the proliferation and death were not revealed in regucalcin-overexpressing RKO cells, and regucalcin overexpression depressed AHR signaling linked to CYP1A1 expression. Thus, AHR signaling suppresses the growth of colorectal cancer cells, suggesting a role as a novel targeting molecule for colorectal cancer.

Keywords: aryl hydrocarbon receptor, 2, 3, 7, 8-tetrachlorodibenzo-*p*-dioxin, TCDD, cell proliferation, cell death, colony formation, RKO cells, carcinogenesis

INTRODUCTION

Intestinal homeostasis is maintained by complex interactions between intestinal microorganisms and the gut immune system, and dysregulation of gut immunity may lead to inflammatory disorders and tumorigenesis [1]. Cross-talk between epithelial cells and stromal cells, such as leukocytes and fibroblasts, is considered to be essential for tumorigenesis and cancer progression [1]. The adenocarcinoma colorectal cancer is the predominant malignancy found in the colon and rectum, and it has been proposed to arise from a small subpopulation of self-renewing tumor stem cells located within the tumor microenvironment [1, 2]. Colorectal cancer is the third most common cancer diagnosed in the developed world [3, 4]. The average 5-year survival rate remains poor at 55% [4]. Colorectal cancer represents a heterogenous group of diseases, and its prognosis remains poor in spite of the development of novel therapeutic strategies [5-8]. The molecular classification of colorectal cancer is important [5-9], and its characterization of novel biomarker targets may lead to prolonged survival in colorectal cancer [10].

The aryl hydrocarbon receptor (AHR) is a ligand-activated transcription factor belonging to the family of basic helix-loop-helix Per-Arnt-Sim (6HLHPAS) transcription factors [11, 12]. AHR forms a heterodimer with the AHR nuclear translocator (ARNT), which is transcriptionally active after binding to xenobiotic responsive elements [11, 12]. The AHR was initially discovered through its binding to the polychlorinated aromatic hydrocarbons such as 2, 3, 7, 8-tetrachlorodibenzo-p-dioxin (TCDD) and polychlorinated biphenyls (PCBs), and polycyclic aromatase hydrocarbons, such as benzo[a]pyrene (B[a]P), and polychlorinated biphenyls (PCBs) [11, 12].

Numerous AHR ligands, as an AHR agonists, have been identified including synthetic and environmental chemicals, naturally occurring dietary and endogenous compounds [13-18]. AHR signaling, which is regulated via various factors, appears to play a crucial role in the regulation of diverse cellular and biological processes [19]. The canonical target genes for AHR are cytochrome P450 isoforms (CYP1A1, CYP1A2 and CYP1B1), which are implicated in the metabolism of xenobiotics and endogenous compounds, including eicosanoids [20, 21]. AHR signaling-dependent pathway is also involved in the process of chemically-induced toxicity and carcinogenesis through the production of free radicals and conversion of pro-carcinogens to ultimate genotoxic carcinogens via metabolism by these enzymes [20, 21]. Moreover, the xenobiotic and ligands of AHR are linked to various toxicities and pathologies in humans, leading to toxic processes, such as tumor promotion, immunosuppression and teratogenicity with disorder of the fine homeostatic regulations of cell functions [22-26].

The physiological function of AHR in the absence of exogenous ligand may be different from its toxicological role after binding of exogenous ligand [27]. Mice expressing a constitutively active AHR showed enhanced development of liver tumors in a model of hepatocarcinogenesis [28]. Notably, AHR signaling may also possess tumor suppressor activities in liver [29], and it may serve to adjust liver repair and regeneration and to block tumorigenesis by modulating stem-like cells and β-catenin signaling [30, 31]. We recently demonstrated that treatment with TCDD at comparatively low levels suppresses proliferation and stimulates the death of human liver cancer HepG2 cells *in vitro*, and that these effects are mediated through mechanistic pathways involving in AHR signaling activity and other-related signaling factors [32].

The AHR has been detected and characterized in human colon adenocarcinoma cells including RKO cells [33-35], and has been shown to regulate the expressions of CYP1A1 [36] and CYP1A2 [37] in colorectal cancer cells *in vitro*. The role of AHR thus has been reported in colon cancer cells [38]. Of note, the AHR suppressed intestinal carcinogenesis in $Apc^{Min/+}$ mice after natural ligand treatment *in vivo* [39]. Moreover, the AHR is associated with tumor prevention by regulating gut immunity in normal intestinal tissues, and it is involved in growth suppression of tumor cells of $Apc^{Min/+}$ mice [16]. Thus, the AHR may play a suppressive role in the development of colorectal cancer. However, the regulatory role of AHR signaling in the proliferation and death of human colorectal cancer cells is poorly understood. We investigated this matter in RKO colorectal cancer cells *in vitro*. We have demonstrated that TCDD treatment suppresses the growth and proliferation and stimulates death of RKO cells, via AHR signaling [40]. Our findings suggest that the activation of AHR signaling plays a suppressive role in the development of human colorectal cancer, revealing a potential novel role of AHR as a target molecule for this disease.

AN AHR AGONIST SUPPRESSES THE GROWTH OF RKO CELLS

We investigated whether the aryl hydrocarbon receptor agonist suppresses human colorectal cancer cells *in vitro*. 2, 3, 7, 8-Tetrachlorodibenzo-*p*-dioxin (TCDD) (>99.99% purity) was dissolved in dimethylsulfoxide (DMSO) and stored in the dark at -20°C until use. We used RKO human colorectal cancer epithelial cells originating from a male adult patients with colorectal carcinoma and obtained from the American Type Culture Collection. RKO cells were suitable as a transfection host, and they were cultured in Dulbecco's Modification of Eagle's Medium (DMEM) with 4.5 g/L glucose, L-glutamine and sodium pyruvate and antibiotics (100 µg/mL penicillin and 100 µg/mL streptomycin; P/S) containing 10% fetal bovine serum (FBS). First, we investigated the effects of TCDD on colony formation of RKO cells *in vitro*. RKO cells were seeded into 6-well dishes at a density of 1×10^3/well, and cultured in DMEM containing 10% FBS, 1% P/S, and 1% fungizone under 5% CO_2 at 37°C in the presence of either vehicle (1% DMSO) or TCDD (1 or 10 nM) for 5 days, when visible clones formed on the plates [41]. This culture was used less cells in a larger well. The dishes were washed with PBS (2 ml, 3 times) and fixed with methanol (0.5 ml per well) for 20 min at room temperature, and then washed 3 times with PBS. The colonies were stained with crystal violet [41]. Crystal violet solution (0.5%, in 20% methanol) was added to the fixed cells for 30 min. Thereafter, stained cells were washed 5 times with PBS. The plates were air-dried for 2 hours at room temperature. The colonies containing more than 50 cells were counted under a microscope. Data were represented as numbers of colonies per well. RKO cells were cultured in the presence of TCDD (1 or 10 nM) for 5 days when visible clones were formed on the plates. The number of colonies with over 50 nuclei was suppressed by treatment with TCDD (1 or 10 nM).

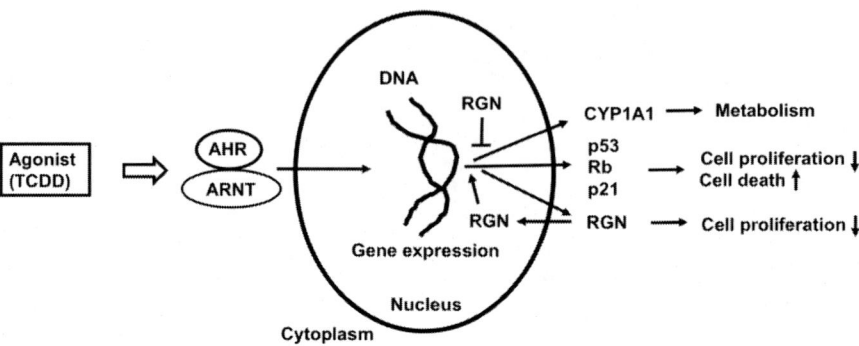

Figure 1. Schematic diagram of the mechanistic link between 2, 3, 7, 8-tetrachlorodibenzo-p-dioxin (TCDD), AHR, CYP1A1, regucalcin (RGN), and other molecules in RKO human colorectal cancer cells. TCDD activates AHR signaling by binding to the AHR nuclear translocator (ARNT). The complex is translocated into the nucleus and regulates expression of various genes. Agonist (TCDD)-activated AHR signaling enhances expression of various genes including CYP1A1, RGN, and p53, Rb, and p21, which is a suppressor of the growth of tumor cells. Overexpressed RGN regulates suppresses the pathways of AHR signaling linked to CYP1A1, leading to inhibition of metabolic pathway. Furthermore, overexpressed RGN enhances the expressions of p53, Rb, and p21, which is increased via TCDD-activated AHR signaling, revealing a potential suppressive effect of cell proliferation and stimulatory effect of cell death. This Figure was listed from Ref. [40].

Moreover, treatment with TCDD was found to exhibit suppressive effects on the proliferation of RKO cells *in vitro* [40]. The RKO cells (1 x 10^5/ml per well) were cultured using a 24-well plate in DMEM (containing 10% FBS, 1% P/S, and 1% fungizone) in the presence of either vehicle (1% DMSO) or TCDD (0.1-100 nM) under 5% CO_2 and 37°C for 3 or 7 days. In separate experiments, RKO cells (1 x 10^5/ml per well) were cultured in DMEM containing 10% FBS, 1% P/S and 1% fungizone with or without either vehicle (1% DMSO) or TCDD (1, 10 or 100 nM) with or without TCDD (10 nM) for 3 days. Cells were then detached from each culture dish to determine cell number. To detach cells in each well, culture dishes were incubated for 2 min at 37°C with a solution (0.1 ml per well) of 0.05% trypsin plus EDTA in Ca^{2+}/Mg^{2+}-free PBS, and then cells were detached through pipetting after the addition of DMEM (0.9 ml) containing 10% FBS and 1% P/S [42].

The medium containing the suspended cells (0.1 ml) was mixed with 0.1 ml of 0.5% trypan blue staining solution. The number of viable cells with viability were counted under a microscope using a Hemocytometer plate and a cell counter. For each dish, we took the average of two counts. Cell number is presented as number per well of plate. First, to determine the effect of TCDD on cell growth, RKO cells were cultured in the presence of TCDD (0.01-100 nM) for 3 or 7 days. The cells reached to subconfluence on culturing for 3 days and to confluence after 4-7 days of culture in 24-well plates. Cell growth was suppressed by treatment with TCDD (0.1-100 nM). Thus, treatment with TCDD was found to exhibit suppressive effects on the proliferation of RKO cells *in vitro* [40].

AN AHR AGONIST STIMULATES THE DEATH OF RKO CELLS

Next, we investigated whether the AHR agonist impacts the death of RKO cells *in vitro*. RKO cells (1 x 10^5/ml per well) were cultured using a 24-well plate in DMEM (containing 10% FBS, 1%P/S, and 1% fungizone) in the absence of TCDD for 3 days. On reaching subconfluence, the cells were cultured in the presence of either vehicle (1% DMSO) or TCDD (0.1-100 nM), with or without the caspase-3 inhibitor (10 µM) either vehicle or CH223191 (1 or 10 µM) for 24 hours [40].

In separate experiments, the RKO-wild type cells or transfectants (1 x 10^5/ml per well) were cultured in DMEM containing 10% FBS, 1% P/S and 1% fungizone in the absence of TCDD for 3 days. On reaching subconfluence, the cells were cultured in the presence of either vehicle (1% DMSO) or TCDD (1, 10 or 100 nM) with or without TCDD (10 nM) for 24 hours. Cells were then detached from each culture dish to determine cell number. Treatment with TCDD (0.1-100 nM) led to decrease of attached cells, indicating that cell death is induced. In separate experiences, on reaching to subconfluence after culture for 3 days, the cells were cultured in the presence of a caspase-3 inhibitor (10 μM) simultaneously with TCDD [40]. The decrease in cell number caused by TCDD (1 or 10 nM) was eliminated by the treatment with the inhibitor of caspase-3.

The activation of caspase-3 induces DNA fragmentation related to apoptotic cell death. The TCDD-induced cell death might be likely due at in least partly to activation of caspase-3, which is known to induce DNA fragmentation related to cell death [40].

AHR SIGNALING MEDIATES TCDD'S EFFECTS ON THE PROLIFERATION AND DEATH OF RKO CELLS

To characterize an involvement of AHR signaling in the revelation of the TCDD-induced suppression of proliferation and stimulation of death of RKO cells, we used 2-methyl-2*H*-pyrazole-3-carboxylic acid (2-methyl-4-*o*-tolylazo-phenyl)-amide (CH223191), as an inhibitor of AHR signaling [43].

Treatment with CH223191 did not have a significant effect on the proliferation or death of RKO cells. The suppressive effect of TCDD (10 nM) on the proliferation and the stimulatory effect of TCDD (10 nM) on the death of RKO cells were both significantly affected by CH223191 (1 or 10 nM) [40]. Whereas the effects of TCDD on cell proliferation were not completely blocked by the inhibitor, although the stimulatory effects of TCDD on cell death was entirely prevented. These findings demonstrate that the effects of TCDD on the proliferation and death of RKO cells are at least partly mediated by AHR signaling.

TCDD ENHANCES THE LEVELS OF PROTEINS LINKED TO TUMOR SUPPRESSION IN RKO CELLS

Furthermore, we investigated whether TCDD treatment impacts the expression levels of intracellular signaling and key transcription factors linked to AHR signaling using western blot analysis [40]. RKO cells were plated in 100 x 21 mm dishes at a density of 1 x 10^6 cells/dish in 10 ml of DMEM containing 10% FBS, 1% P/S, and 1% fungizone, and then cultured in the presence of either vehicle (1% DMSO) or TCDD (10 nM) for 3 days. The cultured cells were washed three times with cold PBS and removed from the dish by scraping in cell lysis buffer supplemented with inhibitors of protease and protein phosphatase. The lysates were then centrifuged at 17,000 g, at 4°C for 10 min, to prepare the cytoplasmic and endoplasmic reticulum fractions.

The protein concentrations of the supernatants were determined using the Bio-Rad Protein Assay Dye with bovine serum albumin as standard. The supernatant was stored at -80°C until use. Samples of 40 micrograms of supernatant protein per lane were separated by SDS polyacrylamide gel electrophoresis (12%, SDS-PAGE), and transferred to nylon membranes for immunoblotting with specific antibodies. Polyclonal AHR antibody sheep IgG was obtained from R&D SYSTEMS. Antibodies to other signaling proteins, including CYP1A1, NF-κB p65, β-catenin and p53, were obtained from Santa Cruz Biotechnology, Inc., and Ras, β-actin, Rb, and p21 were obtained from Cell Signaling Technology [40]. Rabbit anti-regucalcin antibody was obtained from Abcam. Membranes were incubated with each primary antibody overnight at 4°C, followed by horseradish peroxidase-conjugated secondary antibody. Three blots from independent experiments were scanned on an Epson Perfection 1660 Photo scanner, and bands quantified using Image J software.

To determine the mechanism of TCDD's action, we first demonstrated that the AHR and CYP1A1 proteins are present in RKO cells [40], consistent with previous studies showing that the corresponding mRNAs expressed in these cells *in vitro* [34, 35]. TCDD treatment caused a decrease in AHR levels and an elevation of CYP1A1 levels in the cytosol including endoplasmic reticulum of RKO cells [40]. TCDD treatment has been shown to enhance the translocation of cytoplasmic AHR into the nucleus and increases CYP1A1 expression [11, 12, 32].

Of note, TCDD treatment also elevated the levels of NF-κB p65 and β-catenin, which are transcription factors linked to cell signaling, and also increased the levels of p53, Rb, p21, and regucalcin, which are suppressors of tumor cell growth [44, 45]. In addition, regucalcin has been shown to suppress the growth of RKO cells [46]. TCDD treatment did not change the level of Ras, which acts upstream in Akt signaling. β-Catenin has been reported to increase regucalcin expression in HepG2 cells *in vitro* [47]. It has also been reported that p53 modulates Hsp90 ATPase activity, which is implicated in AHR-dependent activation of gene expression [48]. These molecules may be partly involved in mediating the effects of TCDD on the proliferation and death of RKO cells. Schematic diagram of the mechanistic link between AHR agonist (TCDD), AHR, CYP1A1, and other molecules in RKO human colorectal cancer cells is shown in Figure 1.

CONCLUSION

Human colorectal cancer is the third most common cancer diagnosed, but the average 5-year survival rate remains poor at 55%, in spite of the development of novel therapeutic strategies [3-8]. Characterization of novel biomarker targets may ultimately lead to the prolongation of survival of colorectal cancer patients [9]. As described in this chapter, we have demonstrated that the treatment of TCDD, an agonist of AHR, suppresses the growth and proliferation and stimulates death of RKO human colorectal cancer cells. These effects of TCDD were found to be diminished in the presence of CH223191, an inhibitor of AHR signaling [43], indicating that TCDD's effects are at least partly mediated through the AHR signaling pathway. Our findings thus suggest that the activation of AHR signaling plays a suppressive role in the development of human colorectal cancer cells. Thus, the treatment with TCDD, an agonist of AHR signaling, suppresses the growth of human colorectal cancer cells and stimulates their death, via AHR signaling, probably as the result of stimulation of manifold molecules in regulating various signaling pathways. Targeting AHR signaling may cause an anti-tumor effect *in vivo*, suggesting a new strategy for cancer therapy.

REFERENCES

[1] Medema JP, Vermeulen I (2011) Microenvironmental regulation of stem cells in intestinal homeostasis and cancer. *Nature* 474:318-326.

[2] Porter MG, Stoeger SM (2017) A typical colorectal neoplasms. *Surg Clin N Am* 97:641-656.

[3] American Cancer Society. Cancer facts & figures 2016. Atlanta (GA): *American Cancer Society*; 2016.

[4] Siegel RI, Miller KD, Jemal A (2016) Cancer statics, 2016. *CA Cancer J Clin* 66:7-30.

[5] Brenner H, Kloor M, Pox CP (2014) Colorectal cancer. *Lancet* 383:1490-1502.

[6] Alnabulsi A, Murray GI (2016) Integrative analysis of the colorectal cancer proteome; potential clinical impact. *Expert Rev Proteomics* 13:917-927.

[7] Alnabulsi A, Swan R, Cash B, Alnabulsi A, Murray GI (2017) The differential expression of omega-3 and omega-6 fatty acid metabolizing enzymes in colorectal cancer and its prognostic significance. *Brit. J Cancer* 116:1612-1620.

[8] Carini F, Mazzola M, Rappa F, Jurjus A, Geagea AG, Kattar A AL, Bou-Assi T, Jurius R, Damiani P, Leone A, Tomasello G (2017) Colorectal carcinogenesis: Role of oxidative stress and antioxidants. *Anticancer Research* 37:4759-4766.

[9] Colussi D, Brandi G, Bazzoli F, Ricciardiello L (2013) Molecular pathways involved in colorectal cancer: implications for disease behavior and prevention. *Int J Mol Sci* 14: 16365-16385.

[10] Kudryavtseva AV, Lipatova AV, Zaretsky AR, Moskalev AA, Fedorova MS, Rasskazova AS, Shibukhova GA, Snezhkina AV, Kaprin AD, Alekseev BY, Dmitriev AA, Krasnov GS (2016) Important molecular genetic markers of colorectal cancer. *Oncotarget* 7: 53959-53983.

[11] Hankinson O (1995) The aryl hydrocarbon receptor complex. *Annu. Rev. Pharmacol Toxicol* 35:307-340.

[12] Hankinson O (2012) Role of coactivators in transcriptional activation by the aryl hydrocarbon receptor. *Arch. Biochem Biophys* 433:379-386.

[13] Denison MS, Nagy SR (2003) Activation of the aryl hydrocarbon receptor by structurally diverse exogenous and endogenous chemicals. *Annu Rev Pharmacol Toxicol* 43: 309-334.

[14] Nguyen LP, Bradfield CA (2008) The search for endogenous activators of the aryl hydrocarbon receptor. *Chem Res Toxicol* 21:102-116.

[15] Ronnekleiv-Kelly SM, Nukaya M, Diaz-Diaz CJ, Megna BW, Carney PR, Geiger PG, Kennedy GD (2016) Aryl hydrocarbon receptor-dependent apoptotic cell death induced by the flavonoid chrysin in human colorectal cancer cells. *Cancer Lett* 91-99.

[16] Ikuta T, Kurosumi M, Yatsuoka T, Nishimura Y (2016) Tissue distribution of aryl hydrocarbon receptor in the intestine:

Implication of putative roles in tumor suppression. *Exp Cell Res* 343:126-134.

[17] Pastorkova B, Vrzalova A, Bachleda P, Dvorak Z (2017) Hydroxystilbenes and methoxystilbenes activate human aryl hydrocarbon receptor and induce CYP1A genes in human hepatoma cells and human hepatocytes. *Food Chem Toxicol* 103: 122-132.

[18] Safe S, Lee SO, Jin UH (2013) Role of the aryl hydrocarbon receptor ligands in carcinogenesis and potential as a drug target. *Toxicol Sci* 135:1-16.

[19] Mulero-Navarro S, Fernandez-Salguero PM (2016) New trends in aryl hydrocarbon receptor biology. *Front Cell Dev Biol* 4:45. doi:10.3389/fcell.2016.00045. eCollection.

[20] Stejskalova L, Pavek P (2011) The function of cytochrome P450 1A1 enzyme (CYP1A1) and aryl hydrocarbon receptor (AhR) in the placenta. *Curr Pharm Biotechnol* 12: 715-730.

[21] Nukaya M, Moran S, Bradfield CA (2009) The role of the dioxin-responsive element cluster between the Cyp1a1 and Cyp1a2 loci in aryl hydrocarbon receptor biology. *Proc Nat Acad Sci USA* 106:4923-4928.

[22] Pierre S, Chevallier A, Teixeira-Clerc F, Ambolet-Camoit A, Bui LC, Bats AS, Fournet JC, Fernandez-Salguero P, Aggerbeck M, Lotersztajn S, Barouki R, Coumoul X (2014) Aryl hydrocarbon receptor-dependent induction of liver fibrosis by dioxin. *Toxicol Sci* 137:114-124.

[23] Wu D, Nishimura N, Kuo V, Fiehn O, Shahbaz S, Van Winkle L, Matsumura F, Vogel CF (2011) Activation of aryl hydrocarbon receptor induces vascular inflammation and promotes atherosclerosis in apolipoprotein E-/-mice. *Arterioscler Thromb Vasc Biol* 31: 1260-1267.

[24] Brito JS, Borges NA, Esgalhado M, Magliano DC, Soulage CO, Mafra D (2017) Aryl hydrocarbon receptor activation in chronic kidney disease: role of uremic toxins. *Nephron* 137: 1-7.

[25] Esser C (2016) The aryl hydrocarbon receptor in immunity: tools and potential. *Methods Mod Biol* 1371: 239-257.

[26] Murray IA, Patterson AD, Perdew GH (2014) Aryl hydrocarbon receptor ligands in cancer: friend and foe. *Nat Rev Cancer* 14: 801-814.

[27] Barouki R, Coumoul X, Fernandez-Salguero PM (2007) The aryl hydrocarbon receptor, more than a xenobiotic-interacting protein. *FEBS Lett* 581:3608-3615.

[28] Moennikes O, Loeppen S, Buchmann A, Andersson P, Ittrich C, Poellinger L, Schwarz M (2004) A constitutively active dioxin/aryl hydrocarbon receptor promotes hepatocarcinogenesis in mice. *Cancer Re*s 64:4707-4710.

[29] Fan Y, Boivin GP, Knudsen ES, Nebert DW, Xia Y, Puga A (2010) The aryl hydrocarbon receptor functions as a tumor suppressor of liver carcinogenesis. *Cancer Res*70:212-220.

[30] Mathew LK, Simonich MT, Tanguay RL (2005) AHR-dependent misregulation of Wnt signaling disrupts tissue regeneration. *Biochem Pharmacol* 77:714-720.

[31] Jackson DP, Li H, Mitchell KA, Joshi AD, Elferink CJ (2014) Ah receptor-mediated suppression of liver regeneration through NC-XRE-driven p21 Cip1 expression. *Mol Pharmacol* 85: 533-541.

[32] Yamaguchi M, Hankinson O (2018) 2, 3, 7, 8-Tetrachlorodibenzo-*p*-dioxin suppresses the growth of human liver cancer HepG2 cells *in vitro*: Involvement of cell signaling factors. *Int J Oncol* 53:1657-1666.

[33] Harper PA, Prokipcak RD, Bush LE, Golas CI, Okey AB (1991) Detection and characterization of the Ah receptor for 2, 3, 7, 8-tetrachlorodibenzo-*p*-dioxin in the human colon adenocarcinoma cell line LS180. *Arch Biochem Biophys* 290:27-36.

[34] Megna BW, Carney PR, Nukaya M, Geiger P, Kennedy GD (2016) Indole-3-carbinol induces tumor cell death: function follows form. *J Surg Res* 204:47-54.

[35] Megna BW, Carney PR, Depke MG, Nukaya M, McNally J, Larsen L, Rosengren RJ, Kennedy GD (2017) The aryl hydrocarbon receptor as an antitumor target of synthetic curcuminoids in colorectal cancer. *J Surg Res* 212:16-24.

[36] Wohak LE, Krais AM, Kucab JE, Stertmann J, Ovreba S, Scidel A, Ohillips DH, Arlt VM (2016) Carcinogenetic polycyclic aromative hydrocarbons induce CYP1A1 in human cells via a p53-dependent mechanism. *Arch Toxicol* 90:291-304.

[37] Li W, Haper PA, Tang B-K, Okey AB (1998) Regulation of cytochrome P450 enzyme by aryl hydrocarbon receptor in human cells. CYP1A2 expression in the LS180 colon carcinoma cell line after treatment with 2,3,7,8-tetrachlorodibenzo-*p*-dioxin or 3-methylcholanthrene. *Biochem Pharmacol* 56:599-612.

[38] Xie G, Raufman J-P (2015) Role of the aryl hydrocarbon receptor in colon neoplasia. *Cancers* 7:1436-1446.

[39] Kawajiri K, Kobayashi Y, Ohtake F, Ikuta T, Matsushima Y, Mimura J, Petterson L, Pollenz RS, Sakaki T, Hirokawa T, Akiyama T, Kurosumi M, Poellingere L, Kato S, Fujii-Kuriyama Y (2009) AHR suppresses intestinal carcinogenesis in Apc$^{Min/+}$ mice with natural ligand. *Proc Nat Acad Sci* 106:13481-13486.

[40] Yamaguchi M, Hankinson O (2019) 2, 3, 7, 8-tetrachlorodibenzo-*p*-dioxinsuppresses the growth of human colorectal cancer cells *in vitro*: Implication of the aryl hydrocarbon receptor signaling. *Int J Oncol* 54:1422-1432.

[41] Fang Z, Tang Y, Fang J, Zhou Z, Xing Z, Guo Z, Guo X, Wang W, Jiao W, Xu Z and Liu Z: Simvastatin inhibits renal cancer cell growth and metastasis via AKT/mTOR, ERK and JAK2/STAT3 pathway. *PLoS One* 17:8:e62823. doi: 10.1371/journal.pone. 0062823, 2013.

[42] Wang K, Li Y, Jiang YZ, Dai CF, Fatankar MS, Song JS, Zheng J (2013) An endogenous aryl hydrocarbon receptor ligand inhibits proliferation and migration of human ovarian cancer cells. *Cancer Lett* 340:63-71.

[43] Yamaguchi M, Osuka S, Murata T (2018) Prolonged survival of colorectal cancer patients is associated with higher regucalcin gene expression: Overexpressed regucalcin suppresses growth of human colorectal carcinoma cells *in vitro*. *Int J Oncol* 53:1313-1322.

[44] Choi EY, Lee H, Dingle RWC, Kim KB, Swanson HI (2012) Development of novel CH223191-based antagonists of the aryl hydrocarbon receptor. *Mol Pharmacol* 81:3-11.

[45] Tsurusaki Y, Yamaguchi M (2004) Role of regucalcin in liver nuclear function: Binding of regucalcin to nuclear protein or DNA and modulation of tumor-related gene expression. *Int J Mol Med* 14: 277-281.

[46] Yamaguchi M (2013) Role of regucalcin in cell nuclear regulation: involvement of as a transcription factor. *Cell Tissue Res* 354:331-341.

[47] Yamaguchi M, Osuka S, Murata T (2018) Prolonged survival of colorectal cancer patients is associated with higher regucalcin gene expression: Overexpressed regucalcin suppresses growth of human colorectal carcinoma cells *in vitro*. *Int J Oncol* 53:1313-1322.

[48] Nejak-Bowen KN, Zeng G, Tan X, Cieply B, Monga SP (2009) Beta-catenin regulates vitamin C biosynthesis and cell survival in murine liver. *J Biol Chem* 284:28115-28127.

[49] Kochhar A, kopelovich L, Sue E, Guttenplan JB, Herbert B-S, Dannenberg AJ, Subbaramaiah K (2014) p53 modulates Hsp90 ATPase activity and regulates Aryl hydrocarbon receptor signaling. *Cancer Prev Res* 7:596-606.

In: Colorectal Cancer ISBN: 978-1-53616-598-2
Editor: Masayoshi Yamaguchi © 2020 Nova Science Publishers, Inc.

Chapter 4

SURGICAL APPROACH TO RECTAL CANCER

Jelena Petrovic Sunderic[*], MD, PhD*

Department for Coloproctology, University Clinic for
Digestive Surgery, 1st Surgical Clinic, Clinical Center of Serbia,
Belgrade, Serbia

ABSTRACT

Until recently surgery was the only mean of rectal cancer treatment and was not entirely successful in advanced cases. The development of the oncologic agents and radiotherapeutic approaches have given justified hope even for those patients. Nevertheless, the principles of surgery have remained the same, since so far the achieved "gold standard" in rectal cancer surgery, based on total mesorectal excision within the strict anatomic borders, has shown the best immediate and late postoperative results, quality of life and the lowest recurrence rate. New technologies, like laparoscopic and robotic surgeries, are not offering oncologic benefits compared to the open approach, but have immediate postoperative advances. They are becoming more widely accepted both by the surgeons and patients, but are still on trial due to specific considerations. Apart from the radical surgeries, in some cases palliative

---

[*] Corresponding Author's E-mail: jelapetrovic@gmail.com.

procedures are unavoidable, and the aforementioned new oncological advancements can convert inoperable into operable cases.

Keywords: rectum, cancer, surgery, operation, prognosis, quality, assessment, neoadjuvant treatment

INTRODUCTION

Colorectal cancer is one of the most common malignancies in the world with a high incidence of mortality and morbidity, and more than 50% of lesions are found in the distant portions of the colon, that rectum belongs to. Apart from being a relatively common location of malignant and premalignant lesions, rectum requires a special surgical approach due to its anatomy that is also gender specific. Therefore, certain knowledge, experience and skills are necessary in this field of surgery, which is already gaining its independence throughout the world.

The base of the rectal cancer surgery is total mesorectal excision (TME) and it is a procedure that brings adequate lymphadenectomy along with preservation of defecatory, urinary and sexual functions. Depending on the location—mainly distance from the anal verge and involvement of surrounding structures—rectal cancer treatment can have an appropriate approach, involving sphincter-sparing procedure, abdominoperineal resections or transection of the mesorectum.

Development of oncology, like chemo and radiotherapy, has brought more options in rectal cancer treatment. In some cases the combined therapy could lead to the disappearance of the tumor, but mostly, not always, to the decrease in its size and stage. In patients who had the therapy prior to surgery extra care and experience are necessary during operation, since the neoadjuvant (preoperative) treatment does not only influence tumorous cells but also normal tissue, altering the anatomy and quality of tissues.

In locally advanced tumors, sometimes, in spite of neoadjuvant therapy conducted, extensive surgical procedures must be performed and are tailored for each case. Those may include multi-visceral resections of the involving structures, that in some cases include small intestine, abdominal and pelvic walls, urinary bladder, vagina, uterus, ovaries, prostate, sacrum etc. Each of these extensive operations have a goal to remove the tumor entirely, achieve adequate lymphadenectomy with derivation of excretions (stool, urine), and maximally preserve bodily functions.

Development of new technologies, like laparoscopy and robotic surgery, offer certain advances in rectal cancer treatment, allowing better visualization and approach along with the possibility of transanal expression of the specimen, but requiring training, experience and the knowledge of possible complications specific for this field of surgery.

ANATOMIC CONSIDERATION

Rectum is the straight terminal part of the digestive tube. It extends from the sigmoid colon at the point of sacral promontory, following the curve of the sacrum and coccyx and extending further to its wider section, rectal ampulla, after which it ends by anal canal. It varies in length according to the built of the person, and it usually measures around 15 cm above the anal canal, which is about 3-4 cm in length itself. Its proximal part is in the greater pelvic and belongs to the abdominal cavity. It is covered by peritoneum anteriorly, while the lower part is situated in the lesser pelvic extraperitoneally, surrounded by other pelvic structures. In female pelvis it is anteriorly in close relation with vagina, creating a rectovaginal septum, and uterus and ovaries. In males, there are seminal vesicles, prostate and urethra in front of it along with the urinary bladder. The rectovesical septum in males is called Denonvillier's fascia and it is a very important surgical landmark that represents a fascia that extends from the Douglas pouch, the lowest point of the abdominal cavity.

Rectum has very distinguished macroscopic and radiologic features. As an extension of the colon, it is characterized by loss of haustrae, since taeniae coli blend at the point of rectosigmoid junction giving rise to longitudinal muscles that surround the rectum from all sides along its entire length.

Blood supply to the rectum is dual and very reach. Its upper supply is from the extension of the inferior mesenteric artery (AMI), called superior rectal artery. The lower portions are supplied by the internal iliac artery, directly through middle rectal arteries or via internal pudendal arteries (inferior rectal arteries).

Venous drainage corresponds to arterial supply, so the superior part drains into superior rectal vein that is continued by the inferior mesenteric vein, while the lower part is drained by internal pudendal veins and further to the internal iliac veins. Since the superior rectal veins drain into the portal venous system, and the lower part through the internal iliac veins into the systemic circulation, this is an important area of portocaval anastomosis that can explain hematogenic way of spreading of distant metastases to various organs skipping liver.

The lymphatic drainage follows the circulatory pathways and also drains into inferior mesenteric and internal iliac nodes.

Innervation of the rectum is both sympathetic and parasympathetic. The sympathetic innervation comes from the inferior hypogastric plexus, while the parasympathetic is derived from S2-4 nerves that run with pelvic splanchnic nerves to join the inferior hypogastric plexus. The sensory fibers are stimulated by distention of the rectum and they follow the path of the parasympathetic nerves. These nerves are very important for the maintenance of normal sexual, defecatory and urinary functions. Sympathetic and parasympathetic systems act as a unique system in the process of urinary and sexual regulation. In men, sacral parasympathetic fibers innervate cavernous bodies, leading to erection. Injury to this plexus leads to impotence. Sympathetic fibers innervate vasa deferens, prostate, urethra, internal urethral sphincter and control the expression of the semen from the seminal vesicles to the urethra. Activation of this system along with the activation of somatic innervation of ischiocavernosus and bulbospongiosus muscles results in ejaculation. Its injury results in loss of or retrograde ejaculation due to the loss of the internal urethral sphincter innervation. In women, parasympathetic fibers control the vascular engorgement of the clitoris and the vagina, along with the control of transudation of vaginal fluid, which together with secretions from the Bartholin's glands provide adequate vaginal lubrication. Damage to this plexus results in vaginal dryness and dyspareunia. Innervation of the urinary bladder comes from these two systems. Sympathetic fibers innervate base of the bladder, while detrusor muscle is controlled by the parasympathetic fibers. Damage of the parasympathetic fibers causes urinary retention, while rarely seen isolated injuries of the sympathetic system lead to urinary incontinence [1-12]. The male sexual dysfunction is present in around 10-35% of cases after rectal cancer surgery, and in women between 3-57% [13-15]. At the same time urinary dysfunction is reported in 4-27% of cases [16].

About half of all the lesions in the colon that can lead to cancer are found in its distant parts, sigmoid and rectum. Along with its specific position in the pelvis, surgery of the rectal cancer is quite challenging and requires extensive training and experience in order to remove the tumor radically without causing morbidity. Various surgeons at the end of 19th and beginning of the 20th century had realized that the surgery of rectal cancer must be extensive. The mortality was high and quality of life after the surgery was pore. The abdominoperineal resection (APR) or amputation of the rectum was the first widely accepted procedure as an oncologic standard in this pathology. It was independently performed by several surgeons without knowing about each other's work, but it is mostly known as Miles procedure, after Ernest Miles, the surgeon whose work was published by Lancet in 1908 [17]. Later on, Henri Hartmann, a French surgeon, performes a modified operation in which he closes rectum distally from the tumor, at the level of pelvic diaphragm and forms end colostomy. This surgery is known as Hartmann's procedure and is also in use nowadays [18]. During the 50s of the previous century Dixon adopts and improves the technique of sphincter preservation and anastomosis [19]. Only 3 decades later an English surgeon, Richard Heald, improves and promotes anterior resections of the rectum with the concept of the total mesorectal excision (TME), which is still a gold standard in rectal cancer surgery. This considers the division of the rectum with the tumor with en-block lymphadenectomy and resection through the embryologic structures in order to completely excise mesorectum and preserve pelvic nerves. This way the local recurrence rate was lowered from more than 50% to even less than 10% [20].

TREATMENT OF THE RECTAL CANCER

Rectal cancer nowadays has a multidisciplinary approach, while only a few decades ago surgery was the only reliable treatment. Different protocols exist that with more or less success incorporate pre and postoperative therapies into the treatment. Introduction of radiotherapy (RT) as a preoperative treatment through Dutch and Swedish trials has improved the results of modern surgery and those studies had shown the decrease in the incidence of local recurrence that had dropped to only 2.4% and 8% respectively. These were the first trials in which all stage tumors were submitted to neoadjuvant RT, but further follow-up of those patients had led to cognition of severe adverse effects of radiotherapy. Today only advanced cancers are submitted to preoperative radiotherapy, and that includes tumors of T3 and T4 stage or any stage with extensively involved lymph nodes (N2) or mesorectal tumor deposits. Radiotherapy is combined with chemotherapeutic agents in order to increase the local effect on the tumor. This is called chemoradiotherapy (CRT). Nowadays, the uniformly accepted multidisciplinary approach in locally advanced rectal cancer without detectable distant metastases involves a preoperative (so-called neoadjuvant chemoradiation – NCRT) which consists of about 45-50Gy divided into 20-25 fractions with chemopotentiation achieved by addition of Capecitabine, the chemotherapeutic agent, at the beginning and the end of the treatment period. This dose is determined by radiation oncologists and physicists. Six to eight weeks after the completion of NCRT the reevaluation should be made in order to determine the tumor response to therapy and plan future surgery or follow up. In case of the presence of a locally advanced tumor, distant metastasis, pore response to radiotherapy and/or presence of tumor residue after the surgery, patients should receive additional chemotherapy. The chemo, radio, or combined therapy applied after the surgery or as an additional treatment to tumors with initially pore response is called adjuvant therapy. The decision of the necessity to apply adjuvant therapy is also decided by the multidisciplinary team [21, 22].

OVERVIEW OF DIAGNOSTIC PROCEDURES

In order to minimize adverse effects of the therapy, it is crucial to make the accurate diagnosis and staging of the tumor. It is important for surgeons to make an adequate estimate before the surgery.

Apart from the laboratory investigations, that give us information on overall state of the organism, care should be taken to determine whether the patient is anemic (that could mean that he was probably occultly bleeding from the tumor over a longer period of time, but also that he might have another condition that should be brought to the attention), along with the levels of basic tumor markers (CEA and CA 19-9) that are not very reliable in primary diagnostics, but can be useful in the further follow up after the treatment.

Rectal examination can give us information about the location of the tumor, its mobility and relations to the surrounding structures and the anal canal. Digital rectal examination, or "rectal toucher," can give quite accurate information to an experienced surgeon, but only in the lower third of the rectum. Some studies of radiotherapy's direct influence on the tumor have included the surgeon's estimate of the response to therapy based on digital rectal examination as one of the important parameters, along with imaging studies. These parameters consider the presence of the scar tissue at the sight of the irradiated tumor, its firmness or elasticity, mobility and ulceration detection [23].

Rigid rectoscopy is an endoscopic examination that can accurately give us important information about the position of the tumor and its distance from the anal verge. Although sometimes the tumor may be voluminous and/or obstructive, it is important to do a complete colonoscopy whenever possible in order to exclude synchronous tumor in the colon that can occur in about 3-4% of cases [24].

MRI of the pelvis is a standard imaging examination in rectal cancer staging. The new and improved, high-resolution MRI of the rectum, can give us the most accurate estimate of the tumor stage. It offers the possibility to clearly magnify the part of the image we are interested in and give us a better insight of the depth of invasion to the mesorectum and its fascia, anal sphincters, vascular structures, surrounding organs and involvement of the lymph nodes. It is a highly sensitive method that is used also in the estimation of tumor response to previous therapy, which is harder to do due to tissue changes under the influence of neoadjuvant therapy (Figure 1 A, B) [25].

Local stage of the tumor can be estimated by endorectal ultrasound, a much cheaper method that requires an experienced practitioner since it is quite subjective. This is the best method to distinguish between T1 and T2 tumors, while it is not so exact when it comes to advanced stages and lymph node involvement due to the limited visual field it offers. In order to make an exact estimate of the extension of the illness, it is important to perform imaging of the abdomen and thorax in order to detect any possible metastatic deposits. CT and MRI are mostly used for that purpose and are superior to chest radiography and abdominal ultrasonography. [26]

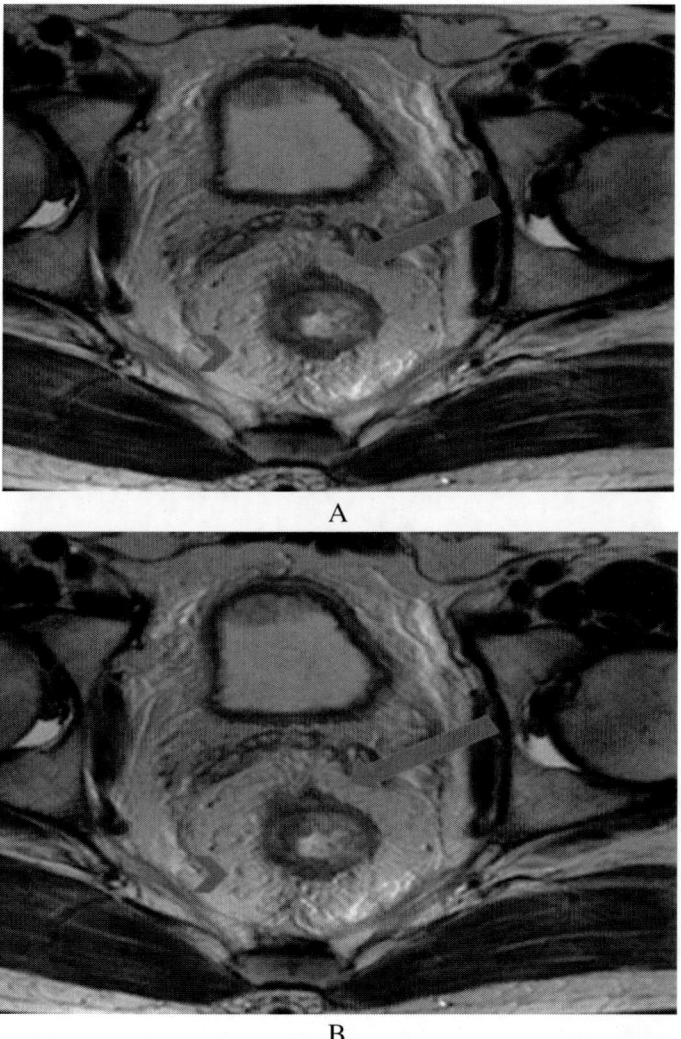

Figure 1. A: An MRI before CRT showing the tumor that does not involve CRM (arrow) and a positive lymph node (arrowhead). B: MRI after CRT showing incomplete response of the tumor (arrow) and a suspicious residue in the lymph node (arrowhead).

SURGERY

Surgery has always been the only therapeutic option that gives immediate results. An adequately operated patient who was accurately diagnosed and staged can be cured by surgery alone. Of course, this considers early stage cancer with minimal or absent lymphonodal involvement. Neoadjuvant and adjuvant therapies offer solutions to the ones with advanced tumors, but principles of surgery do not change much accordingly.

Surgery is planned with respect to the stage of the tumor, its distance from the anal verge and involvement of surrounding structures. This estimate is based on imaging and physical findings. It is very important for a surgeon to be familiar with every kind of diagnostics because he is the one to plan and perform the procedure. Based on this estimate we can roughly divide the surgical treatment into palliative and radical.

Palliative Surgery

There are several reasons to perform palliative procedures, and it involves very advanced, inoperable and obstructive tumors in patients who are not in a condition to sustain major surgery. These procedures do not lead to healing of the patient, but can, to some extent, improve the quality of life. These procedures include diversion stomas, stenting of the tumor, palliative radiotherapy and cryotherapy.

Diversion stomas can be performed in several different ways and do not necessarily have to be the final surgical treatment. In patients who are potentially operable, they are protection from the obstruction during neoadjuvant CRT. In case further surgery is planned, it is important to also plan the use of stoma. Some authors recommend diversion colostomy, while others consider sigmoidostomy as more convenient for the patient. Ileostomy does not have to be reversed during the radical surgery, but used as a protection of anastomosis, while sigmoidostomy usually has to be mobilized in order to achieve the length of the colonic transplant. The disadvantage of ileostomy is threatening dehydration, so many surgeons nowadays aim to create diversion coecostomies and transversostomies as a compromising solution with satisfying results [27].

Not so long ago the diagnostic and imaging procedures were not so sophisticated and widely available. It was not uncommon, and this still happens especially in emergency cases due to the obstruction or fracture of the tumor, that the patient gets operated on without adequate staging. In those cases, even at the attempt of radical surgery, sometimes the end colostomy is the best solution. In emergency cases of obstructive tumors that are in the proximal rectum within the abdominal cavity and not susceptible to radiotherapy, or in peritonitis due to the leakage at the sight of the tumor, surgeons tend to do as much as possible to save lives and are frequently forced to remove the tumor with creation of end colostomy. In cases of peritonitis with fractured tumor it has to be removed as a source of infection, while in tumors that cause obstructions there is a great discrepancy in the size of the lumen for the potential anastomosis that is not a favorable factor. Therefore many surgeons tend to make a diversion stomas in order to lower the pressure in the colon and achieve shrinkage of the colonic wall that would allow the creation of anastomosis during the radical surgery, once the diagnostics and the potential neoadjuvant treatment are completed.

Other palliative treatments include palliative RT and cryotherapy that offer shrinkage of the tumore with the consequential widening of the lumen, while self-expanding stents keep the lumen open at the level of the tumor.

Radical Surgical Procedures

Radical procedures are the ones by which the tumor is entirely removed along with its lymphatics and vascular pedicle, and clearance of all resection margins is verified by a pathologist. According to the position of the tumor, especially the distance from the anal verge, the preservation of the anal sphincter is planned.

The patient is placed in a supine position with legs spread for the better exposure of the pelvis and perineum, the so-called Lloyd-Davis position. The surgery starts with mobilization of the left colon and splenic flexure. In about 1% of cases, the injury of the spleen happens, more often in open surgery usually due to the inadequate traction of the splenocolic ligament that leads to tears of the splenic capsule. In only 15% of cases, the spleen can be preserved, but splenectomy is mostly unavoidable [28].

After the mobilization of the left colon and separation of mesocolon from the retroperitoneum by dissecting through Toldt's fascia, the vascular stamp, that includes AMI and vein, is divided. AMI should be ligated about 1-2 cm away from the aorta in order to preserve preaortic sympathetic nerves. Due to the possibility of colonic marginal artery interruption at the level of the splenic flexure (a point of mesenteric arterial connection between the superior and inferior mesenteric arteries, also known as meandering mesenteric artery or arcus Riolani) it is advisable to preserve the left colic artery, the brunch of the inferior mesenteric artery. The neglect of this issue can lead to the insufficient vascularization of the anastomosis and its leakage.

The next step is the division of colon at the level of sigmoid and further mobilization of the proximal rectum down to the point of the pelvic diaphragm. The posterior part is initially mobilized by cutting through the posterior side of the mesorectal fascia and following the curvature of the sacral bone.

It is important to remember that the superior hypogastric plexus lies over and bifurcates at the level of the sacral promontory and dissection through the accurate layer preserves the damage of these nerves.

In tumors of the proximal and middle rectum, it is proven to be safe to transect the rectum about 5 cm below the lower edge of the tumor. These anastomoses are mostly located intraperitoneally above the ampulla recti and do not require diversion stomas. Apart from that, very good functional results are seen in mesorectal transections.

In tumors at or below the peritoneal reflection the lateral dissection extends from the exposed posterior side of the mesorectum, with preservation of the hypogastric nerves that come from both sides as "errigent pillars" [29].

In sphincter-sparing operations, the excision of the most caudal part of the mesorectum is crucial in nerve preservation and achievement of oncologic radicality. This is achieved by the division of the rectosacral fascia (also known as Waldeyer's fascia that originates from S2-S4 and divides mesorectum into superior and inferior compartments), instead of being misled by it and leaving inferior mesorectal lymphatic and fatty tissue behind. Following of the right plane would lead to interspictheric space that completes the adequate excision of the mesorectum [30].

The border of the anterior resection should be an extension of the plane obtained by the lateral dissection. This phase is very demanding in the means of nerve preservation. It is very important to include peritoneal reflection (Douglas pouch) in the specimen, since the important landmark, Denonvillier's fascia, represent its extension into the lesser pelvis (Figure 2). This fascia presents the border between the rectum and the anterior structures (prostate and seminal vesicles in men and vagina in women). Respectful dissection through this layer helps in the preservation of the vegetative nerves. In men, at the point of the prostate, the Denonvillier's fascia is adherent to the prostate, so it should be divided transversally at this level [31].

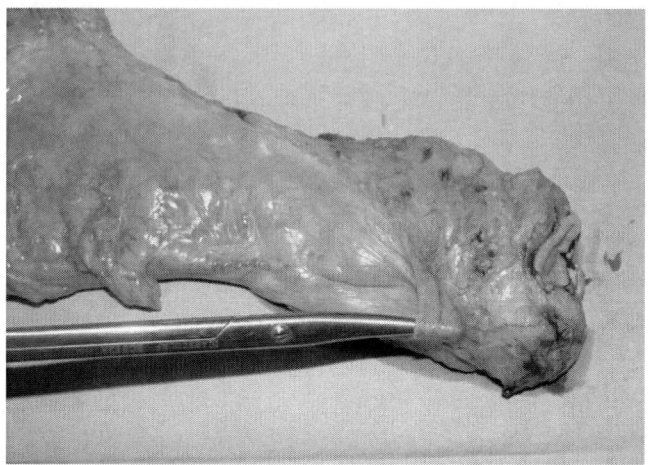

Figure 2. Douglas pouch excised and removed with the specimen.

In very low tumors with involvement of anal sphincters, abdominoperineal resections (APR) are performed. It considers resection of the rectum and anus with the creation of end colostomy. In order to preserve vegetative nerves and avoid conning of the specimen at the sphincter level (narrowing of the width of the specimen at the sphincter level, thus inadequately resecting the tissue), some authors advise 'face down" reposition of the patient for the perineal part of the surgery. The excision of the coccyx is a standard part of this procedure and it allows better visualization of the prostate and the neurovascular bundles, along with the adequate excision of the levator muscles (Figure 3 A, B).

In sphincter-sparing surgeries (SSP) the anastomosis can be created between colon and anus or colon and rectum. In anastomosis with the anus, it is important to make a small reservoir that mimics the ampulla recti and allows the stool to be held in for a while since there is a discrepancy in the size of the lumen at the level of the sigmoid colon and ampulla recti. This reservoir can be created as a colonic pouch or a simple side to end anastomosis, whose blindly closed end forms a pouch. Extensive studies showed that there is no significant difference in functional results a year after these types of procedures [32].

Most of the surgeons advise diversion creation in sphincter-sparing procedures. The main role of the stoma is a diversion of intestinal content away from the anastomosis, especially in cases of anastomotic leakage. If this complication happens, the presence of stoma can prevent reoperation that would lead to taking down of anastomosis and other life-threatening complications, and allow conservative treatment by transanal drainage that could lead to healing of the anastomosis. In case of leakage without stomas, emergency laparotomy must be performed to treat peritonitis and prevent sepsis [33].

Special considerations are taken in tumors of early and very advanced stages. The tumor does not have to be voluminous to be aggressive and give regional and/or distant metastases in an early stage or can be voluminous, involving surrounding structures, but without secondary deposits.

When it comes to voluminous, locally aggressive tumors ultraradical surgeries can be performed, like pelvic exenteration, which considers block resection of the rectum, prostate, seminal vesicles and urinary bladder in men (total pelvic exenteration) or vagina, uterus and ovaries in women (posterior pelvic exenteration) along with the extended lymphadenectomy. When the urinary bladder is involved in the resection it is necessary to create the urine diversion too. This can be achieved by creating ileal conduit along with the colostomy, or double barrel wet colostomy as a single reservoir for the excretions. It is, of course, more comfortable to have only one pouch instead of two, but because of the high incidence of pyelonephritis in wet colostomy after a year from surgery, it is advisable to separate the diversions in patients with longer life expectancy [34].

When tumor involves also omentum, small intestine, uterus, and/ or other organs, multivisceral en block resections are advised in order to avoid the spillage of the malignant cells and further dissemination [35].

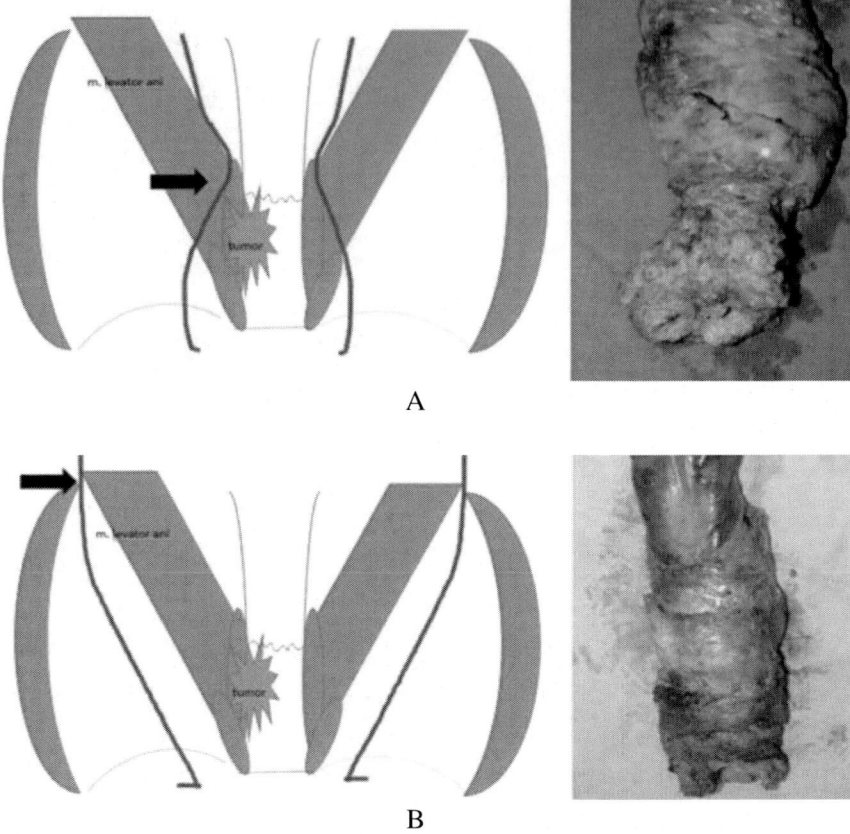

Figure 3. A: Conning effect at the level of anal sphincters (arrow) with the photo of a specimen, B: No conning effect with the complete excision of levators and the photo of a specimen (arrow).

Transanal Excision

Although transanal excisions and TEM (transanal endoscopic mucosectomy) are not advisable, in selected cases of early rectal tumors without the involvement of the lymph nodes those can be adequate treatments in preservation of the quality of life. These patients must be closely monitored afterwards and quickly treated if any sign of recurrence occurs [36].

Watch 'n' Wait

Radiotherapy has offered the possibility to avoid major surgery in cases of complete response (CR). In several prospective studies, these patients were closely monitored during the follow-up and the assessment was made based on digital rectal examination, endoscopic evaluation and imaging studies (MRI, CT, PET scan). Special protocols were developed for this "watch and wait" approach. About 10% of patients develop clinical complete response and most of them would not have distant metastasis within three years, along with about 70% with the same disease-free survival. The major problem in these protocols is the assessment of the lymph node involvement, since the imaging criteria of nodal involvement is 1cm in size, and after CRT they may shrink to 3mm and still have viable malignant cells that cannot be accurately detected by standard imaging techniques [37, 38].

Laparoscopic and Robotic Surgery

New technologies, like laparoscopic and robotic surgery, have offered some advantages over the open surgery for rectal cancer. Newest studies have shown that the laparoscopic surgery can offer better visualization of the pelvis, better immediate postoperative functional results and a lower rate of surgical site infections, although the principles of surgery remain completely the same. The preparation for surgery is slightly more extensive than in the conventional approach, requiring better purgation of guts, but fits better in the fast track surgical mode of recovery, offering benefits of early ambulation. Oncologic results do not differ much from the ones in open surgery. Therefore, in skilful hands, the laparoscopic approach can be state of the art in rectal cancer surgery. Robotics is much more expensive than laparoscopy and have the equivalent functional and oncologic results, but offer greater comfort to the surgeon that many consider priceless, since a well-trained surgeon is still more important than any technological achievement so far. Apart from that, a lower rate of conversion and better exposure of the vegetative nerves is noticed but is also associated with the longer operative time than the conventional laparoscopic approach [39, 40, 41].

In order to achieve objective results, the assessment of surgery is additionally made by pathologists. The inspection of the specimen must show the shiny, intact mesorectal fascia covering the rectal specimen, the presence of levators on the APR specimen and vascular pedicle, along with the evaluation of the distant and lateral clearance from the tumor. Apart from the evaluation of the quality of surgical performance, accurate response to CRT can also be made. The pathology report points towards the patients who would benefit from adjuvant therapy [42].

Additional evaluation of the surgical performance, along with the consequences of the additional therapy is further made by the patient himself. That considers urinary, defecatory and sexual functions (dryness of vagina in women, impotence, ejaculation, retrograde ejaculation in men, etc.), as well as a subjective feeling of disfigurement, sadness, insecurity, discomfort in public places, etc.), troubles with colostomy pouch and other similar issues. Quality of life has been the focus of many recent studies, and the results are improving with the development of new technologies and surgical techniques along with the consciousness of the importance of vegetative nerve preservation, in order to prevent sexual and urinary dysfunctions.

CONCLUSION

Surgery of the rectum can result in sphincter preservartion (with or without the formation of temporary diversion of the intestinal content) or in removal of rectum and anus with permanent stoma creation, according to the stage of the tumor and its distance from the anal verge.

Due to its specific anatomic position and surrounding structures in the pelvic, rectal cancer requires precise initial diagnostics and treatment tailored for the patient. Upper portion of the rectum is covered by peritoneum and is easily accessible by abdominal approach, but the lower part is situated in the lesser pelvic extraperitoneally and adheres to surrounding organs and structures.

Good knowledge of pelvic anatomy and precise surgical technique are necessary for successful rectal cancer surgery, which includes complete extraction of tumor according to the oncologic parameners (en block excision of the tumor with surrounding lymphatics) and preservation of sympathetic and parasympathetic nerves that should insure good quality of life (preservation of digestive, sexual and urinary functions). In order to achieve all these goals it is always required to make precise preoperative staging of the tumor and find possible metastasis.

In cases of locally advanced and/or distal and metastatic tumors it is necessary to make a multidisciplinary approach that may lead to a decision to include other modalities of treatment, like radio and chemotherapy.

The preoperative (neoadjuvant) therapy in cases of advanced and tumors with distant localization can enable higher quality surgery regarding oncologic (downsizing and downstaging of the tumor and lymphatics) and functional (sphincter and pelvic nerve preservation) results. These treatments are known to turn inoperable cases into operable ones, or even lead to complete tumor eradication (complete response).

In spite of all these scientific and technical achievements, in very advanced cases with surrounding organ involvement sometimes it is necessary to make multiorgan resections and even mutilating operations. In very advanced tumors it is crucial to determine whether an attempt for the radical surgery can give any benefit to the patient or even be harmful, leaving it to palliative or other nonsurgical treatments.

For all these reasons rectal cancer surgery is state of the art in digestive surgery and requires great knowledge, experience, open mind and perfect surgical technique, along with realistic judgement and good collaboration with other specialists as a part of a very complex oncologic treatment.

ACKNOWLEDGMENT

The author thanks for the editing of manuscript by Dr. Pravin J Gupta, MS, FICS, FASCRS, FCS, FAIS, FISCP, Fine Morning Hospital and Research Center, Laxmi Nagar, Nagpur, India.
E-mail: drpjg@yahoo.co.in.

REFERENCES

[1] Krivokapić ZV, Dimitrijević I, Barišić G (2012) Anatomy and Phisiology of the Rectum and Anal Canal (Anatomija i fiziologija rektuma i analnog kanala). In: Krivokapic Z (de) Rectal Cancer (Karcinom rektuma) 1st Ed. Zavod za udžbenike, Belgrade 23-29.

[2] Alasari S, Lim D, Kim NK (2015) Magnetic resonance imaging-based rectal cancer classification: landmarks and technical standardization. *World J Gastroenterol* 14:21:423-431. https://doi: 10.3748/wjg.v21.i2.423.

[3] Wasserman MA, McGee MF, Helenowski IB, Halverson AL, Boller AM, Stryker SJ. (2016) The anthropometric definition of the rectum is highly variable. *Int J Colorectal Dis* 31:189-195. hppts://doi: 10.1007/s00384-015-2458-5.

[4] Dujovny N, Quiros RM, Saclarides TJ (2004) Anorectal anatomy and embryology. *Surg Oncol Clin N Am* 13:277-293.

[5] Brunicardi FC AD, Billiar TR, Dunn DL, Hunter JG, Matthews JB, Pollock RE (2010) Schwartz's Principles of Surgery. 9th ed: McGraw-Hill; p1888.

[6] Wang GJ, Gao CF, Wei D, , Wang C, Meng WJ (2010) Anatomy of the lateral ligaments of the rectum: A controversial point of view. *World J Gastroenterol* 16: 5411–5415.

[7] Moore KL (2014) The pelvis and perineum. Clinically Oriented Anatomy, Lippincott Williams & Wilkins pp. 289-293.

[8] Sobotta J (1972) Atlante di Anatomia. UTET – sansoni Ediziani scientifiche, Firenze.

[9] Netter FH (1989) Atlas of Human Anatomy, 9th printing Ciba Pharmaceuticals Division, Ciba-Geigy Corporation.

[10] Fozard JBJ, Pemberton JH (1998) Applied Surgical Anatomy, Pelvic Contents in Rob - Smith's Operative Surgery.

[11] Nivatvongs S, Gordon PH (2007) Surgical anatomy In Principles and Practice of Surgery for the Colon, Rectum and Anus. Informa Healthcare USA. 3rd Edition. 1-29.

[12] Heald RJ, Moran BJ (1998) Embryology and Anatomy of the Rectum. *Semin Surg Oncol* 15: 66-71.

[13] De Palma GD, Luglio G (2015) Quality of life in rectal cancer surgery: What do the patient ask?. *World J Gastrointest Surg* 7:349-355. https://doi: 10.4240/wjgs.v7.i12.349.

[14] Havenga K1, Maas CP, DeRuiter MC, Welvaart K, Trimbos JB (2000) Avoiding long-term disturbance to bladder and sexual function in pelvic surgery, particularly with rectal cancer. *Semin Surg Oncol* 18:235-243.

[15] Hendren SK, O'Connor BI, Liu M, Asano T, Cohen Z, Swallow CJ, Macrae HM, Gryfe R, McLeod RS (2005) Prevalence of male and female sexual dysfunction is high following surgery for rectal cancer. *Ann Surg* 242:212-223.

[16] Chew MH, Yeh YT, Lim E, Seow-Choen F (2016) Pelvic autonomic nerve preservation in radical rectal cancer surgery:

changes in the past 3 decades. *Gastroenterol Rep* (Oxf) 4:173-185.

[17] Miles WE (1908) A Method Of Performing Abdomino-Perineal Excision For Carcinoma Of The Rectum And Of The Terminal Portion Of The Pelvic Colon. The Lancet. Volume 172, issue 4451, p1812-1813. https://doi.org/10.1016/S0140-6736(00)99076-7.

[18] Hartmann H (1921) Nouveau procédé d´ablation des cancers de la partie terminale du colon pelvien. *Trentième Congrès Francais de Chirurgie* 30: 309-311.

[19] Dixon CF (1948) Anterior resection for malignant lesions of the upper part of the rectum and lower part of the sigmoid. *Ann Surg* 128: 425-442.

[20] Heald RJ, Husband EM, Ryall RD (1982) The mesorectum in rectal cancer surgery-the clue to pelvic recurrence? *Br J Surg* 69: 613-616.

[21] Kapiteijn E, Marijnen CA, Nagtegaal ID, Putter H, Steup WH, Wiggers T, Rutten HJ, Pahlman L, Glimelius B, van Krieken JH, Leer JW, van de Velde CJ; Dutch Colorectal Cancer Group (2001) Dutch Colorectal Cancer Group. Preoperative radiotherapy combined with total mesorectal excision for resectable rectal cancer. *N Engl J Med* 345:638-646.

[22] Folkesson J, Birgisson H, Pahlman L, Cedermark B, Glimelius B, Gunnarsson U (2005) Swedish Rectal Cancer Trial: long lasting benefits from radiotherapy on survival and local recurrence rate. *J Clin Oncol* 23:5644-5650.

[23] Pozo ME, Fang SH (2015) Watch and wait approach to rectal cancer: A review. *World J Gastrointest Surg* 7: 306–312. https://doi: 10.4240/wjgs.v7.i11.306.

[24] King-Yin Lam A, Sze-Yan Chan S, Leung M (2014) Synchronous colorectal cancer: Clinical, pathological and molecular implications. *World J Gastroenterol* 20: 6815–6820. https://doi: 10.3748/wjg.v20.i22.6815.

[25] Battersby NJ1, How P, Moran B, Stelzner S, West NP, Branagan, Strassburg J, Quirke P, Pedersen BG, Gudgeon M, Heald B, Brown G; MERCURY II Study Group (2016) Prospective Validation of a Low Rectal Cancer Magnetic Resonance Imaging Staging System and Development of a Local Recurrence Risk Stratification Model: The MERCURY II Study. *Ann Surg* 263:751-760. https://doi: 10.1097/SLA.0000000000001193.

[26] Oien K, Mjørud Forsmo H, Rosler C, Nylund K, Waage JE, Pfeffer F (2019) Endorectal ultrasound and magnetic resonance imaging for staging of early rectal cancers: how well does it work in practice? *Acta Oncol* 8:1-6. https://doi: 10.1080/0284186X.2019.1569259.

[27] Klink CD1, Lioupis K, Binnebösel M, Kaemmer D, Kozubek I, Grommes J, Neumann UP, Jansen M, Willis S (2011) Diversion stoma after colorectal surgery: loop colostomy or ileostomy? *Int J Colorectal Dis* 26:431-436. https://doi: 10.1007/s00384-010-1123-2.

[28] Masoomi H1, Carmichael JC, Mills S, Ketana N, Dolich MO, Stamos MJ (2012) Predictive factors of splenic injury in colorectal surgery: data from the Nationwide Inpatient Sample, 2006-2008. *Arch Surg* 147:324-329. https://doi: 10.1001/archsurg.2011.1010.

[29] Heald B (2008) Autonomic nerve preservation in rectal cancer surgery - the forgotten part of the TME message a practical "workshop" description for surgeons. *Acta Chir Iugosl* 55:11-116.

[30] Garcia-Armengol J, Garcia-Botello S, Martine-Soriano F, Roig JV, Liedo S (2008) Review of the Anatomic Concepts in Relation to the retrorectal Space and Endopelvic Fascia: Waldeyer's Fasciaand the Rectosacral Space. *Colorectal Dis* 10:298-302. https://doi: 10.1111/j. 1463-1318.2007.01472.x.

[31] Lindsey I, Guy RJ, Warren BF, Mortensen NJ (2000) Anatomy of Denonvilliers' fascia and pelvic nerves, impotence, and implications for the colorectal surgeon. *Br J Surg* 87:1288-1299.

[32] Markovic V, Dimitrijevic I, Barisic G, Krivokapic Z (2015). Comparison of Functional Outcome of Colonic J-Pouch and Latero-Terminal Anastomosis in Low Anterior Resection for Rectal Cancer. *Srpski Arhiv Za Celokupno Lekarstvo* 143: 158-161. https://doi: 10.2298/SARH1504158M.

[33] Zuri A, Murrell MD, Michael J, Stamos MD (2006) Reoperation for Anastomotic Failure. *Clin Colon Rectal Surg* 19: 213–216. doi: 10.1055/s-2006-956442.

[34] Salgado-Cruz L, Espin-Basany E, Vallribera-Valls F, Sanchez-Garcia J, Jimenez LM, Marti-Gallostra M, Garza-Maldonado A (2014) Double barreled wet colostomy: initial experience and literature review. *ScientificWorldJournal* 2014:961409.

[35] Hoffmann M, Phillips C, Oevermann E, Killaitis C, Roblick UJ, Hildebrand P, Buerk CG, Wolken H, Kujath P, Schloericke E, Bruch HP(2012) Multivisceral and standard resections in colorectal cancer. *Langenbecks Arch Surg* 397:75-84. doi: 10.1007/s00423-011-0854-z. Epub 2011 Oct 4.

[36] Baral J (2018) Transanal endoscopic microsurgical submucosa dissection in the treatment of rectal adenomas and T1 rectal cancer. *Coloproctology* 40:364-372.

[37] 2017 European Society of Coloproctology (ESCP) collaborating group. (2018) Evaluating the incidence of pathological complete response in current international rectal cancer practice: the barriers to widespread safe deferral of surgery. *Colorectal Dis* 20 (Suppl): 6:58-68. https://doi: 10.1111/codi.14361.

[38] Habr-Gama A, Sabbaga J, Gama-Rodrigues J, São Julião GP, Proscurshim I, Bailão Aguilar P, Nadalin W, Perez RO (2013) Watch and wait approach following extended neoadjuvant chemoradiation for distal rectal cancer: are we getting closer to anal cancer management? *Dis Colon Rectum* 56:1109–1117.

[39] Petrovic J, Antic S, Krivokapic ZV (2012) Preparation of the patient for colorectal surgery (Priprema bolesnika za operaciju

kolona I rektuma) In: Krivokapic Z (de) Rectal Cancer (Karcinom rektuma) 1st Ed. Zavod za udžbenike, Belgrade 163-175.

[40] Małczak P, Mizera M, Torbicz G, et al. (2018) Is the laparoscopic approach for rectal cancer superior to open surgery? A systematic review and meta-analysis on short-term surgical outcomes. *Wideochir Inne Tech Maloinwazyjne* 13:129-140. https://doi: 10.5114/wiitm.2018.75845.

[41] Nozawa H1, Watanabe T1 (2017) Robotic surgery for rectal cancer. *Asian J Endosc Surg* 10:364-371. https://doi: 10.1111/ases.12427. Epub 2017 Sep 26.

[42] Song SB, Wu GJ, Pan HD, Yang H, HuML, Li Q, Yan QX, Xiao G (2018) The quality of total mesorectal excision specimen: A review of its macroscopic assessment and prognostic significance. *Chronic Dis Transl Med* 4:51-58. https://doi:10.1016/j.cdtm. 2018.02.002.

ABOUT THE EDITOR

Masayoshi Yamaguchi
Adjunct Professor, University of Hawaii Cancer Center,
University of Hawaii at Manoa

Masayoshi Yamaguchi, PhD, IOM, FAOE, DDG, DG, is Adjunct Professor, Cancer Biology, University of Hawaii Cancer Center, University of Hawaii at Manoa (2019-), Visiting Professor, Department of Pathology and Laboratory Medicine, David Geffen School of Medicine, University of California, Los Angeles (UCLA) (2017-2019); Adjunct Professor, Emory University School of Medicine, Atlanta, USA (2013-2016); Visiting Professor, Emory University School of Medicine (2007-2011); Professor, Graduate School of Nutritional Sciences, University of Shizuoka, Japan (1992-2007). Dr. Yamaguchi discovered two novel proteins (genes), which were named regucalcin and RGPR-p117. Since 1974, Dr. Yamaguchi published over 550 English articles in professional journals with peer-review. Dr. Yamaguchi serviced as Editorial Board Members in 90 Journals thus far. Dr. Yamaguchi received "The 2017 Albert Nelson Marquis Lifetime Achievement Award" Marquis Who's Who, USA), Member of World Academy of Sciences.

INDEX

#

6-dichloro-1-β-D-ribofuranosylbenzimidazole, 37
8-Tetrachlorodibenzo-*p*-dioxin, 55, 64

A

abdominal and pelvic walls, 69
ACF, 16
acid, 5, 10, 17, 18, 47, 62
acidic, 24
adaptive immune response, 8
adenocarcinoma, ix, 21, 31, 33, 45, 47, 52, 54, 64
adhesion, 9, 15, 18
adjustment, 5
adrenal gland, 44
advancements, xi, 68
adverse effects, 72, 73
agonist, x, 51, 55, 57, 60, 61
AHR nuclear translocator, x, 51, 53, 56
algae, viii, 1, 6
algorithm, 34
alters, 27

ampulla, 69, 79, 80
anastomosis, 70, 72, 77, 78, 80, 81
anatomy, 68, 85, 86, 87
angiogenesis, vii, 15, 18, 27
antioxidant, 5, 6, 9, 21, 25
antitumor, 11, 21, 25, 26, 28, 38, 43, 65
antitumor agent, 38, 43
apoptosis, vii, viii, 2, 4, 7, 8, 9, 10, 11, 12, 13, 14, 15, 16, 17, 20, 22, 23, 24, 26, 27, 46
apoptotic pathways, 14
apoptotic protease activating factor 1, 7
arabinose, 8, 10, 13
aromatic hydrocarbons, 53
arrest, viii, ix, 2, 9, 11, 12, 13, 17, 20, 25, 26, 32, 38, 39, 49
arteries, 70, 78
aryl hydrocarbon receptor, x, 51, 52, 53, 55, 62, 63, 64, 65, 66
assessment, 68, 83, 84, 91

B

bacteria, 3, 15, 28
barriers, 90
base, 68, 71

basement membrane, 3
Bay K 8644, 37, 40
beneficial effect, 18
benefits, xi, 67, 83, 88
biochemistry, 6
biological activities, 6, 19
biological processes, 14, 53
biosynthesis, 66
bladder cancer, 22
bone, 5, 22, 44, 46, 78
bone marrow, 5, 22, 44
breast cancer, ix, 31, 33, 43, 44, 46
butyrate, 16, 38, 39, 48

C

Ca^{2+}, 38, 40, 42, 45, 49, 56
Ca^{2+}-dependent kinases, 42
calcium, 5, 32, 38, 42, 45
cancer, v, vii, viii, ix, x, xi, 1, 2, 3, 4, 5, 6, 7, 9, 10, 12, 13, 14, 15, 16, 18, 19, 20, 22, 23, 24, 25, 26, 27, 28, 29, 31, 32, 33, 34, 35, 36, 37, 39, 42, 43, 44, 46, 47, 48, 49, 51, 52, 54, 55, 56, 60, 61, 62, 64, 65, 66, 67, 68, 69, 71, 72, 74, 76, 83, 85, 86, 87, 88, 89, 90, 91, 93
cancer cells, vii, x, 3, 4, 5, 7, 8, 9, 12, 33, 39, 42, 43, 44, 45, 46, 51, 54, 61
cancer suppressor gen, 3
carboxylic acid, 3, 58
carcinogenesis, vii, ix, 10, 31, 33, 35, 44, 46, 47, 52, 53, 54, 62, 63, 64, 65
carcinoma, ix, 17, 25, 32, 36, 48, 55, 65, 66
caspase-3, 7, 10, 12, 14, 16, 40, 57, 58
caspase-3 inhibitor, 40, 57, 58
cDNA, 36, 37, 39, 41, 45
cell cycle, ix, 3, 9, 10, 11, 12, 13, 17, 20, 24, 25, 26, 32, 38, 39, 42, 43, 49
cell death, 11, 14, 26, 32, 37, 40, 43, 50, 52, 56, 58, 62, 64
cell differentiation, 13

cell line, 10, 12, 20, 64, 65
cell proliferation, vii, 7, 10, 15, 23, 25, 26, 32, 37, 38, 39, 40, 42, 43, 46, 47, 48, 49, 52, 56, 58
cell signaling, 46, 60, 64
cellular homeostasis, 14
cellular immunity, 17
chemical structures, 19
chemicals, 6, 53, 62
chemotherapeutic agent, 72
chemotherapy, vii, viii, 1, 4, 5, 6, 22, 73, 85
chemotherapy drugs, viii, 1, 5, 6
chest radiography, 75
classification, viii, x, 33, 51, 53, 86
clinical application, 19
cognition, 72
colitis, 9, 15, 18, 24, 29
colon, viii, 1, 2, 3, 4, 5, 6, 7, 8, 10, 12, 13, 14, 15, 16, 18, 19, 20, 21, 22, 23, 24, 25, 26, 27, 28, 33, 52, 54, 64, 65, 68, 70, 71, 74, 77, 78, 80, 88
colon cancer, viii, 1, 2, 3, 4, 5, 6, 7, 8, 10, 12, 13, 14, 15, 16, 18, 19, 20, 22, 23, 24, 25, 26, 27, 28, 54
colon carcinogenesis, 10
colony formation, ix, x, 32, 37, 44, 52, 55
colorectal cancer, viii, ix, x, xi, 1, 2, 4, 9, 10, 18, 20, 24, 25, 26, 28, 29, 31, 32, 33, 34, 35, 37, 44, 47, 48, 51, 52, 54, 55, 56, 60, 61, 62, 65, 66, 68, 88, 90
colorectal cancer cells, x, 9, 24, 25, 37, 44, 51, 54, 55, 56, 60, 61, 62, 65
colorectal surgeon, 89
colostomy, 72, 76, 77, 80, 81, 84, 89, 90
complex interactions, 52
consciousness, 84
controversial, 87
corolectal cancer, 2
Corolectal cancer, 2
culture, 11, 36, 37, 40, 41, 43, 55, 56, 57
Cyclin D, 18
Cyclin E, 12

Cyclin A1, 4
Cyclin D1, 4
cyclooxygenase 2, 9
CYP1A1, x, 52, 53, 54, 56, 59, 60, 63, 65
CYP1A2, 53, 54, 65
CYP1B1, 53
cytochrome P450 isoforms, 53
cytoplasm, 8, 9

D

database, ix, 31, 34
degradation, 11
dendritic cell, 22
deoxyribonucleic acid, 48
detection system, 41
developed countries, 2
diaphragm, 72, 78
dibucaine, 37, 38, 42
dietary fiber, 5
dimethylsulfoxide, 55
dioxin, 55, 56, 63, 64
diseases, viii, x, 14, 22, 33, 51, 52
disorder, 4, 53
distribution, 25, 62
DNA, 3, 5, 9, 32, 38, 40, 43, 50, 58, 66
DNA damage, 3, 10, 38, 43
DNA fragmentation, 40, 58
DNA repair, 9
down-regulation, 7, 17
drugs, viii, 1, 4, 5, 6, 33
dysplasia, vii

E

electrophoresis, 41, 59
emergency, 77, 81
endothelial cells, 15
enzymes, 32, 47, 53, 62
epidemiology, 2, 3
epidermal growth factor receptor, 4

epigenetic alterations, viii, 33
epithelial cells, 2, 28, 52, 55
epithelial RKO cells, 36
EPS1-1, 17, 18, 19
ERK, 20, 38, 42, 65
errigent pillars, 79
etiology, 1, ii, iii, 3
eukaryotic cell, 11
excision, xi, 67, 68, 72, 79, 80, 82, 85, 88, 91
exopolysaccharide (EPS1-1), 16, 17, 18, 19, 28
exopolysaccharides, 20
extracellular signal-regulated kinas, 38

F

fascia, 69, 74, 78, 79, 84, 89
fatty acids, 3, 7, 15, 16
feces, 16, 18
fibroblasts, 48, 52
fibrosis, 63
formation, ix, x, 12, 14, 32, 37, 44, 52, 55, 84
free radicals, 53
fungi, viii, 1
fungus, 16, 26

G

G1 and G2/M phase cell cycle arrest, ix, 32, 38, 39
G1 phase, 11, 12, 26, 48
G2 phase, 11
galactose, 10, 13, 17
galacturonic acid, 10
gastrointestinal tract, 15
gel, 41, 59
gemcitabine, 22, 37, 38, 43

gene expression, ix, 7, 10, 17, 25, 28, 31, 32, 33, 34, 35, 43, 44, 46, 47, 48, 50, 60, 66
gene therapy, 34, 46
genes, vii, 3, 4, 10, 14, 16, 48, 49, 53, 56, 63, 93
genetic marker, 48, 62
genus, 16
ginseng, 6, 22, 27
glucose, 8, 10, 13, 17, 36, 55
glucosidic linkages, 19
glucuronic acid, 10
glutamine, 36, 55
glycobiology, 6
goblet cells, 18
graduate students, xi
growth, x, 3, 4, 9, 10, 12, 13, 15, 17, 20, 26, 33, 34, 36, 44, 45, 48, 51, 54, 56, 57, 60, 61, 64, 65, 66
gut microbiota, 15, 16, 18, 28

H

haemopoiesis, 27
hair, 5
HCT-116, 7, 11, 12, 17, 23
healing, 76, 81
hematochezia, 18
hepatocarcinogenesis, 54, 64
hepatocellular carcinoma, 33, 44
hepatoma, 39, 43, 48, 49, 50, 63
high fat, 3
homeostasis, 32, 46, 52, 61
hormones, 4
human, viii, ix, x, 1, 2, 7, 9, 10, 12, 13, 14, 15, 17, 19, 21, 22, 23, 24, 25, 26, 27, 28, 31, 33, 34, 35, 36, 37, 39, 42, 43, 44, 45, 46, 48, 49, 51, 54, 55, 56, 60, 61, 62, 63, 64, 65, 66
human subjects, 33, 34
humoral immunity, 17

I

IL-17, 9
IL-1β, 9
IL-2, 17
IL-6, 9, 14, 18
ileostomy, 77, 89
immune system, 52
immunity, 17, 18, 27, 52, 54, 64
immunofluorescence, 38
immunosuppression, 5, 53
immunotherapy, 4, 22
in vitro, viii, ix, x, 1, 6, 11, 14, 17, 18, 19, 32, 33, 34, 36, 37, 39, 43, 44, 46, 47, 48, 51, 54, 55, 56, 57, 60, 64, 65, 66
in vivo, 6, 11, 14, 17, 18, 33, 34, 54, 61
incidence, viii, 2, 3, 14, 68, 72, 81, 90
individual character, 3
induction, 20, 23, 26, 63
inflammation, 5, 63
inhibition, 9, 12, 17, 19, 25, 32, 38, 39, 43, 56
inhibitor, ix, x, 9, 32, 38, 39, 40, 42, 43, 48, 49, 52, 57, 58, 61
inhibitor of AHR signaling, x, 52, 58, 61
intestinal homeostasis, 52, 61
invasion, vii, 2, 9, 15, 18, 24, 26, 27, 29, 74

K

Kaplan-Meier curve, 35
kidney, 5, 39, 50

L

Lactobacillus, 20
laparoscopic surgery, 83
laparoscopy, 69, 83
large intestine, 16

lead, vii, viii, x, 33, 35, 39, 40, 44, 51, 52, 60, 68, 71, 76, 78, 79, 81, 85
leakage, 77, 78, 81
lentinan, 6, 22
lesions, 5, 68, 71, 88
leukocytes, 52
life expectancy, 81
ligand, x, 51, 53, 54, 65
liver, ix, 5, 6, 31, 33, 43, 44, 45, 46, 50, 54, 63, 64, 66, 70
liver cancer, ix, 31, 33, 43, 54, 64
liver damage, 5
lung cancer, 33, 43, 47
lymph, 44, 72, 74, 75, 82, 83
lymph node, 44, 72, 74, 75, 82, 83
lymphocytes, 17

migration, 8, 9, 13, 15, 18, 23, 24, 27, 65
mitochondria, 7, 8
Mitochondrial Apoptotic Pathway, 7
mitogen, 11, 38, 49
mitogen-activated protein kinase, 11, 38, 49
mitogen-activated protein kinases, 11, 49
mitosis, 11
molecular weight, 8, 10, 13, 15, 17, 19
molecules, 7, 33, 42, 56, 60, 61
monosaccharide, 19
morbidity, viii, 68, 71
mortality, viii, 2, 68, 71
mRNA, 10, 35, 48
MST1, 4
mucosa, 3
muscles, 70, 71, 80
mutations, 3, 48

M

M phase, ix, 10, 11, 13, 32, 38, 39, 49
macrophages, 11, 17, 28
magnetic resonance imaging, 89
malignancy, viii, 33, 52
malignant cells, vii, 81, 83
MAPK Signaling Pathway, 11
MAPKs, 11
matrix metallopeptidase 2, 9
matrix metallopeptidase 9, 9
matrix metalloproteinases, 18
mechanisms, viii, 1, 6, 14, 20
medical, xi
medical science, xi
medicine, 6, 19
metastasis, vii, viii, 2, 4, 6, 9, 15, 16, 18, 27, 29, 44, 65, 73, 83, 85
methanol, 37, 55
mice, 13, 15, 16, 17, 18, 21, 22, 23, 25, 28, 54, 63, 64, 65
micrograms, 41, 59
microorganisms, 3, 6, 52
microscope, 37, 38, 55, 57

N

National Academy of Sciences, 28
natural polymers, 6
neoadjuvant treatment, 68, 77
nerve, 79, 84, 85, 87, 89
neurogenetic disorders, 45
neurotoxicity, 5
NF-κB, viii, ix, x, 1, 8, 9, 11, 18, 23, 32, 42, 43, 52, 59, 60
NF-κB p65, ix, x, 9, 32, 42, 43, 52, 59, 60
NF-κB Signaling, 8, 23
nitric oxide synthase, 9
nodal involvement, 83
nuclear transcription factor, 8
nuclei, 43, 55
nucleus, 8, 40, 44, 56, 60

O

obstruction, 76, 77
omega-3, 47, 62
omentum, 81

oncogenes, 4, 44
operation, 2, 68, 71
operations, 69, 79, 85
organs, 70, 74, 81, 85
osteoclastogenesis, x
ovarian cancer, 65
overexpression, ix, x, 4, 24, 32, 40, 42, 44, 46, 47, 49, 50, 52

P

p21, ix, x, 7, 12, 32, 39, 42, 43, 52, 56, 59, 60, 64
p21WAF1/CIP1, 12
p53, ix, x, 4, 7, 9, 10, 12, 17, 18, 24, 32, 42, 43, 52, 56, 59, 60, 65, 66
P53 Apoptosis Pathway, 9
palliative, xi, 67, 76, 77, 85
pathways, 8, 9, 27, 32, 38, 42, 43, 46, 47, 54, 56, 61, 62, 70
pelvis, 69, 71, 74, 78, 79, 83, 87
penicillin, 36, 55
perineum, 78, 87
peritoneum, 69, 85
peritonitis, 77, 81
pharmaceutical, 16
phosphatidylinositol 3-kinase, 38
phosphor-MAPK, 42
phosphor-SAPK/JNK, 42
phosphorylation, 7, 8, 11, 49
PI3K, viii, 1, 13, 27, 38, 49
PI3K/AKT, 13, 27
plasma membrane, 45
polychlorinated biphenyls (PCBs), 53
polysaccharide, 2, 6, 7, 8, 9, 10, 11, 12, 13, 14, 15, 16, 20, 21, 22, 23, 24, 25, 26, 27, 28, 29
Polysaccharides, v, 1, 6, 15, 19, 23, 25, 27
portal venous system, 70
preservation, 68, 72, 78, 79, 82, 84, 85, 87, 89

prevention, viii, xi, 1, 5, 19, 47, 54, 62
prevention and treatment, 4, 19
principles, xi, 67, 76, 83
prognosis, vii, viii, 33, 48, 52, 68
pro-inflammatory, 14
pro-inflammatory cytokines, 14
proliferation, vii, ix, x, 2, 3, 4, 5, 7, 8, 10, 11, 12, 13, 14, 15, 17, 23, 25, 26, 27, 32, 37, 38, 39, 40, 42, 43, 44, 46, 47, 48, 49, 52, 54, 56, 57, 58, 60, 61, 65
prophylactic, 5, 17
prostaglandin, 9
prostate, 69, 71, 79, 80, 81
protein kinases, 11, 32, 38, 42, 49
protein synthesis, 32
proteins, 8, 25, 41, 42, 44, 59, 60, 93
proto-oncogene, 3, 4

Q

quality of life, viii, xi, 1, 6, 67, 71, 76, 82, 85

R

radiation, vii, 73
radical procedures, 78
radio, 73, 85
radiotherapy, viii, 1, 4, 6, 68, 72, 74, 76, 77, 83, 88
Radiotherapy, 6, 72, 83
Ras, ix, x, 32, 42, 52, 59, 60
Rb, ix, x, 7, 32, 42, 43, 52, 56, 59, 60
reactive oxygen, 12, 17, 23
receptor, x, 4, 62, 63, 64, 66
rectal cancer, xi, 67, 68, 69, 71, 73, 74, 83, 85, 86, 87, 88, 89, 90, 91
rectosigmoid, 70
rectum, viii, 2, 33, 52, 68, 69, 70, 71, 74, 77, 78, 79, 80, 81, 84, 85, 86, 87, 88, 90
recurrence, xi, 4, 6, 67, 72, 82, 88

Index

regucalcin, v, ix, x, 31, 32, 33, 34, 35, 36, 37, 38, 39, 40, 41, 42, 43, 44, 45, 46, 47, 48, 49, 50, 52, 56, 59, 60, 66, 93
regulations, 53
repression, 32, 39
resection, 71, 78, 79, 80, 81, 88
response, ix, 2, 10, 19, 73, 74, 75, 83, 84, 85, 90
reticulum, 59, 60
retrograde ejaculation, 71, 84
rgn, 32
Rhizopus, 16, 28, 29
Rhizopus nigricans, 16, 28, 29
rigid rectoscopy, 74
risk factor(s), 3
RKO cell(s), ix, x, 32, 34, 36, 38, 39, 40, 42, 43, 44, 52, 54, 55, 56, 57, 58, 59, 60
RNA, 5, 32, 38, 43, 49
room temperature, 37, 55
roscovitine, 37, 39, 48

S

SAPK/JNK, ix, 32, 42
scar tissue, 74
SDS-PAGE, 41, 59
seminal vesicle, 69, 71, 79, 81
serum, 17, 18, 36, 41, 55, 59
serum albumin, 41, 59
sigmoid colon, 2, 69, 80
signal transduction, 10
signaling pathway, vii, viii, ix, 1, 4, 8, 11, 13, 14, 32, 39, 41, 42, 49, 61
SLA, 89
SLNT, 7
small intestine, 69, 81
sodium, 24, 36, 37, 49, 55
solution, 38, 40, 55, 56, 77
sphincter, 68, 71, 72, 78, 79, 80, 81, 84, 85
sphincter-sparing surgeries, 80
spleen, 17, 78

suppression, ix, 5, 9, 32, 34, 44, 54, 58, 63, 64
surgery, viii, xi, 1, 4, 67, 68, 69, 71, 72, 73, 76, 77, 78, 80, 81, 83, 84, 85, 86, 87, 88, 89, 90, 91
surgical resection, 6
surgical technique, 84, 85, 86
survival, viii, ix, x, 5, 17, 31, 33, 34, 35, 44, 46, 47, 48, 51, 52, 60, 66, 83, 88
survival rate, viii, x, 5, 33, 51, 52, 60
SW480, 10, 12, 14, 27
sympathetic system, 71
synthesis, 5, 32, 43, 48

T

target, vii, 7, 11, 22, 27, 53, 54, 63, 65
techniques, 83
technologies, xi, 67, 69, 83, 84
tetrachlorodibenzo-p-dioxin, x, 51, 52, 53, 64, 65
therapeutic targets, vii, 49
therapy, vii, x, 6, 32, 43, 68, 69, 73, 74, 84, 85
thorax, 74
tissue, 18, 64, 68, 74, 79, 80
TLR4, 9, 11
TNF-α, 8, 9, 17, 18, 40
toxic side effect, 6
transanal endoscopic mucosectomy, 82
transanal excisions, 82
transcription, ix, 8, 14, 17, 31, 32, 41, 42, 43, 46, 49, 53, 59, 60, 66
transcription factors, 42, 43, 53, 59, 60
transfectants, 36, 37, 39, 40, 57
transplantation, 16
treatment, vii, viii, x, xi, 2, 4, 5, 6, 10, 11, 12, 15, 17, 19, 52, 54, 55, 56, 58, 59, 60, 61, 65, 67, 68, 69, 72, 73, 76, 77, 81, 85, 86, 90
trial, xi, 67

tumor, vii, ix, x, 2, 3, 4, 6, 7, 8, 9, 11, 13, 14, 15, 16, 17, 19, 21, 22, 23, 24, 25, 27, 28, 31, 33, 34, 35, 40, 42, 43, 44, 46, 48, 50, 52, 53, 54, 56, 60, 61, 63, 64, 66, 68, 69, 71, 72, 73, 74, 75, 76, 77, 78, 79, 81, 84, 85
tumor cells, x, 3, 4, 7, 11, 13, 15, 52, 54, 56
tumor development, 44
tumor necrosis factor-α, 40
tumors, viii, 5, 33, 54, 69, 72, 74, 76, 77, 79, 80, 81, 82, 85

U

ulceration, 5, 74
ultrasonography, 75
unsaturated fatty acid, 5
urinary bladder, 69, 71, 81
urinary dysfunction, 71, 84
urinary retention, 71
uterus, 69, 81

V

vagina, 69, 71, 79, 81, 84
vascular endothelial growth factor (VEGF), 18

vascularization, 78
visualization, 69, 80, 83

W

water, 8, 11, 12, 13, 23, 37
Western blot, x, 41, 42, 52
wild type, 57
Wnt signaling, 64
Wnt/β-catenin signaling pathway, 14
wortmannin, 37, 38, 42

X

X chromosome, 32

α

α-1,3-fucosyltransferase-VII, 15, 24

β

β-actin, 59
β-catenin, ix, x, 14, 18, 32, 42, 43, 52, 54, 59, 60
β-catenin signaling, 14, 54

Related Nova Publications

PENILE CANCER: CHALLENGES AND CONTROVERSIES

EDITORS: Francisco E. Martins, MD and Miroslav L. Djordjevic, MD, PhD

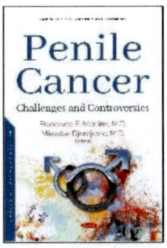

SERIES: Cancer Etiology, Diagnosis and Treatments

BOOK DESCRIPTION: This book will have contributions from world-renowned experts in this field from different continents, providing an international flare and perspective on the recent developments in the field of diagnosis and treatment penile cancer as well as reconstruction of the devastating effects of penile mutilation.

HARDCOVER ISBN: 978-1-53615-950-9
RETAIL PRICE: $230

THE STORY OF HYDRA: PORTRAIT OF CANCER AS A STEM-CELL DISEASE

AUTHOR: Shi-Ming Tu, MD

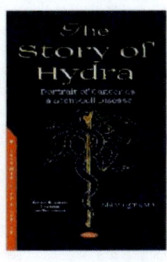

SERIES: Cancer Etiology, Diagnosis and Treatments

BOOK DESCRIPTION: We illustrate that cancer is a multicellular rather than a unicellular process, a cellular rather than a genetic problem, and a stem-cell rather than a somatic-cell disease. We reveal that the incredible resemblance between a cancer cell and a stem cell suggests that they are intimately related.

HARDCOVER ISBN: 978-1-53615-373-6
RETAIL PRICE: $230

To see a complete list of Nova publications, please visit our website at www.novapublishers.com

Related Nova Publications

New Developments in Oncology Research

Editor: Marcos T. Blair

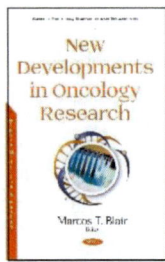

Series: Cancer Etiology, Diagnosis and Treatments

Book Description: In the opening chapter, authors discuss the current literature that describes the application of Palliative Medicine services in advanced cancer, models of Palliative Care delivery by site and mode of practice, cost-effectiveness of early Palliative Medicine referral patterns and national and international Palliative Medicine practice and referral guidelines.

Hardcover ISBN: 978-1-53615-365-1
Retail Price: $160

To see a complete list of Nova publications, please visit our website at www.novapublishers.com